"Sanford's groundbreaking account is meant to offer a powerful message about the endurance of the human spirit and of the body that houses it."

—PN/*Paraplegia News*, May 2006

"Like the best narratives, this journey takes you into new and unexplored realms of meaning. I cried and laughed and ultimately experienced transformational insights about my own life, elucidating not only the physical trials but also travails and triumphs of the soul. From a hard-won understanding of how the body has intelligence and is an aspect of the soul, the author presents us with a new revitalizing vision of what it is to be human."

—Susan Griffin,
author, Pulitzer Prize-nominated *A Chorus of Stones*

"[Sanford's] paralysis has taught him powerful lessons about consciousness, and he shares them with lucidity in this funny but wrenching memoir. Still, it's his story of how he came to embody his grown-up life as a paraplegic—complete with wife, kids, and a job as a yoga instructor—that will truly dare readers to appreciate their own bodies and lives."

—*Yoga Journal*, October 2006

D0062490

"Waking will wake you up, give you a substantial jolt of hope, and change your relationship to the most ordinary actions you take."

—Patricia Weaver Francisco,
author of *Telling: A Memoir of Rape and Recovery*

"This is a riveting, heartbreaking, heart-opening saga . . . His insights are seeds that acquire power and shape over time—months after first reading it, I find myself appreciating his writing and the depth of his thinking more and more."

—Nina Utne,
chair, *Utne* magazine

"It is a 'hero's journey' of separation, initiation, and return. However, the hero of Waking *is profoundly human. He is not larger-than-life, of mythological dimensions, or otherwise a hero to idolize and worship, but is an ordinary human being confronted with extraordinary circumstances."*

—Kristi Swenson-Mendez,
assistant professor of Religious Studies,
Virginia Commonwealth University

Matthew Sanford's remarkable story puts a human face on an alternative healing path. His experience as a patient and his exploration of yoga and paralysis inform and inspire patients, doctors, and rehabilitation professionals alike. He beautifully underscores the limitations of our current medical practices and the necessity for a mind-body-spirit approach to healing and recovery. Matthew is a rising star in the integrative health movement.

—Donna Karan,
chief designer and creative director, Donna Karan International
and founder, Urban Zen Foundation

"This is a beautiful, life-giving book. It reads like poetry and takes the reader inside Matthew Sanford's struggles and insights as a paraplegic and a man, a son, a brother, a husband, and a father. But the "transcendence" of the book's subtitle is not otherworldliness. This is a story of moving gracefully within the limits, tragedies, surprises, and ordinariness of being human and alive."

—Krista Tippet,
Speaking of Faith, American Public Media

"Sanford offers a powerful, honest account of his battle: awakening a spirit within a damaged body."

—*Psychology Today*, August 2006

"On the surface, Matthew Sanford's story makes for terribly gripping reading. But the real reason to pick it up is for the beautiful simplicity with which he describes the mind-body relationship. Through his personal story of healing, he shares inspiring insights for anyone exploring awareness and the essence of life itself."

—Kaitlin Quistgaard,
editor-in-chief, *Yoga Journal*

"Sanford's writing inspires not because of any drama or melodrama connected to loss, but because it awakens us to nonmedical possibilities of healing—discovering ways our minds can connect with our bodies to open windows to wholeness—something disabled and nondisabled alike can embrace."

—*New Mobility magazine*, June 2006

". . . A beautifully written account of his story. It is sobering, with its revelations of just how unbearable human existence can become after such a physical trauma, yet reassuring, through its narrative of how one man can adapt and learn from his own experience what an entire medical establishment had told him not to believe."

—*Minneapolis Star Tribune*, June 2006

WAKING

WAKING

MATTHEW SANFORD

A MEMOIR OF TRAUMA AND TRANSCENDENCE

RODALE

© 2006 by Matthew Sanford

Book design by Christopher Rhoads

Library of Congress Cataloging-in-Publication Data

Sanford, Matthew.
  Waking : a memoir of trauma and transcendence / by Matthew Sanford.
     p.   cm.
  ISBN-13: 978-1-59486-302-8 hardcover
  ISBN-10: 1-59486-302-4 (pbk.) hardcover
  ISBN-13: 978-1-59486-845-0 paperback
  ISBN-10: 1-59486-845-X paperback
  1. Sanford, Matthew. 2. Paraplegics--Biography. 3. Yoga--Health aspects. I. Title.
RC406.P3S26   2006
362.196'8420092--dc22   2006009370

Distributed to the trade by Holtzbrinck Publishers

         14 16 18 20 19 17 15   paperback

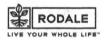

We inspire and enable people to improve their lives and the world around them
For more of our products visit **rodalestore.com** or call 800-848-4735

For William and Paul

Contents

Acknowledgments

I have learned that a book is not written solely by one person. I have a horde of people to thank, and not everyone can be mentioned here. But I am grateful to all of you.

I feel profound gratitude for the revolutionary work of yoga master Sri B.K.S. Iyengar. His inclusive method of yoga has made all of this possible for me. I must also thank my yoga teacher Jo Zukovich and her husband, Mike. Without her steady but gentle and compassionate guidance, I would never have persisted. I am honored to call both of them my friends. I also want to thank any and all yoga teachers, past and present, who have helped me, including Manouso Manos who has taught me in ways I am still figuring out.

I am grateful for all the music that I have listened to while writing this book and, in particular, for the music of the Dave Matthews Band, U2, and Keith Jarrett.

A developing manuscript needs thoughtful readers, and I have had many of them: Kerri Neville, Teri Carter, Susanne Otos, Anna Paulson, Mia Lynch, and especially Larry Lavercome. I also want to thank Nina Utne for her tireless help and ongoing support.

Special thanks goes to Patricia Francisco, who convinced me to write my story as a memoir, who helped me every step of the way, and who showed me how to fall in love with the process of writing. I must also thank my agent, Marly Rusoff, who believed in my work and had the patience to help me mature as a writer. I also want to offer my heartfelt thanks to my editor, Leigh Haber, who had the courage to take a chance on my story and ensured that the best version of *Waking* made its way into the world.

I must also thank my mother, Paula Sanford, who has faithfully listened to her youngest son struggle to articulate his thoughts for the last twenty-seven years. Finally, a special thank you to my wife, Jennifer. She has had to live with this book every day for eight years and is still willing to hug me.

The Mind-Body Relationship

Hope is the dream of a waking man.
—*Aristotle*

There is a difference between seeking and looking for answers. I am not looking for answers. Rather, I seek to appreciate and believe in my experience.

I know what it feels like to leave my body. I learned to do this as a means to survive devastating trauma. At the age of thirteen, I was in a car accident that killed my father and sister. It also pounded my body and left me paralyzed from the chest down. During my first three months in the hospital, leaving my body became a survival skill. I needed to separate from it—otherwise, there was too much pain.

These experiences alone put me in unknown territory when it comes to mind and body. But now add the paralysis that I have lived with for the past twenty-five years. My mental awareness—through a spinal cord injury—was literally knocked out of the lower two-thirds of my body. If someone tickles the bottoms of my feet, my mind does not register a tickling sensation. When my mental awareness reaches downward, below my chest, I cannot make my body move, nor do I feel any sense of control. Instead, I experience a form of silence.

Add to this what I encountered during my initial recovery. While doctors were able to keep me alive, I was not given any tools to reconnect my mind to my paralyzed body. In fact, I was taught that such a connection was no longer possible, that my paralysis (and the silence that came with it) was simply a loss. For the first twelve years after the accident, I believed it.

As I write this book, I am a yoga teacher, and I still get around in a wheelchair. I teach bodies that can stand when I cannot, that can feel things where I do not. This is possible because I have explored a different kind of connection between mind and body. Although I still cannot move my legs—and have no goal to do so—I do feel a heightened level of presence throughout my entire consciousness, including my paralyzed body.

It is a connection that we all share. Most of us, however, have not needed to bring it fully to consciousness. I believe this shared connection has profound implications not just for the shape and quality of our consciousness, but for the aging process, for the experience of trauma, for our approach to disability and rehabilitation, and even for our survival on this planet. By *consciousness,* I mean the sum total of whatever we are—mind, body, spirit, and any other term that aims to describe the totality of our presence. This book is my first attempt to articulate something about our consciousness that has struck me because of my unusual experiences with mind and body.

In principle, my experience is not different from yours. It is only more extreme. If I asked you to stretch the muscles between your ribs or to directly lift your arches, chances are you would have no idea how to proceed. We all live with versions of mind-body disconnection.

My mind-body relationship changed in an instant—the time it took for my back to break. But the changing relationship between mind and body is a defining feature of everyone's life. We are all leaving our bodies—this is the inevitable arc of living. Death cannot be avoided; neither can the inward silence that comes with the aging process.

I now experience a different, more subtle connection between mind and body. It does not require that I flex muscles. It does not dissipate in the presence of increasing inward silence. In fact, this connection depends on it. It does require, however, that I seek more profoundly within my own experience and do so with an open mind. It means that I must reach intuitively into what may feel like darkness.

Two important descriptive terms appear throughout my story: *silence* and *healing stories*. *Silence* is the word I use to describe the empty presence we experience within our experience—between our thoughts, between each other, between ourselves and the world. We feel the silence when we daydream, when we appreciate the beauty of a sunset, or when the love of our life truly walks away. It is an inward sense, often experienced as a longing or an ache. It is a feeling of emptiness and fullness at the same time. The silence is the aspect of our consciousness that makes us feel slightly heavy. It is the source of the feeling of loss, but also of a sense of awe.

A *healing story* is my term for the stories we have come to believe that shape how we think about the world, ourselves, and our place in it. They can be as simple as "Everything happens for a reason" or as sharp as "How come nothing ever works out for me?" Healing stories guide us through good and bad times; they can be both constructive and destructive, and are often in need of change. They come together to create our own personal mythology, the system of beliefs that guide how we interpret our experience. Quite often, they bridge the silence that we carry within us and are essential to how we live.

My story is full of healing stories. They have come from health-care professionals, from my family, from myself, and eventually from the practice of yoga. These stories have profoundly shaped my perceptions of my own body and of how my body and mind interact. They determine whether I see possibilities within the silence of my paralysis or stop at feeling only its limitations. I believe that we all share an inevitable confrontation with an increasing silence. I also believe that our healing stories truly matter.

So I offer my story of mind and body. During my thirteenth year, the silence within my consciousness cracked wide open. My life ever since has attempted to bring this experience to waking.

Part One
Trauma and Separation

1

Early Morning

For the first seven years of my life, my nickname was Jolly—Jolly because my smile, pudgy cheeks, and a potbelly intimated that a giggle was just around the corner.

Some people are born with a smile on their face, and I am one of them. I do not mean this metaphorically. I literally mean that my mouth does not seem to possess the ability to form a frown, like a tongue that cannot curl. Instead, the outer corners of my mouth turn slightly upward, making my default expression a smile. After all that has happened, I am grateful for this fact.

This does not mean that I am particularly upbeat or light-hearted. In fact, my wife, Jennifer, complains that I am unrelentingly serious, especially in the descending moments before sleep. It is then that Jennifer knows to stop reading and extinguish her light. Her eyes close as she utters the words "It's time to lay down, lover."

It is early morning, and I am lying in bed. I am entering the summer that approaches my thirty-ninth birthday. I still have those boyish jolly cheeks, curly light brown hair, and a short beard that is beginning to show hints of gray. In a few hours, I will be teaching my Monday, 9:30 yoga class. As usual, I am not sure what I will teach, but I am hoping for inspiration, a sudden burst of how a particular yoga pose feels. I am looking for a feeling that can bridge the gap between my own paralyzed body and the walking bodies of my students.

Sitting up without disturbing Jennifer's sleep is difficult. I grab the edge of the bed and pull myself over to my right side. As I do, my gaze encounters my wheelchair, like it has for more than a quarter of a century. Even after all this time, I am often surprised to see it sitting quietly at my bedside, waiting not for someone else but for me. In one continuous movement, I swing my legs off the bed and rise to a sitting position. After twenty-five years of paralysis and thirteen years of yoga, my muscles below my chest remain unresponsive to my direct command. I put one hand on the seat of my wheelchair, one hand firmly on the bed, and lift myself onto the main source of my mobility.

I am up early this morning to practice *pranayama,* the yogic art of breathing. I want to finish before my house wakes, before Jennifer's coffeemaker begins to groan, before my son's feet begin to travel across our wooden floors. As I wheel silently down the hallway, I do not feel my feet against my foot pedals, but I do feel a buzz, a hum that travels throughout my entire body, both my paralyzed and unparalyzed body. I gently lower myself down onto our living room rug. It is a transfer that has taken years to perfect—to move as a unified whole, to combine flexing arms and flaccid legs into a single flowing movement.

The morning sunlight beams through our east-facing windows

and creeps across my body. I am lying on two accordion-folded blankets that run along the length of my spine. A third blanket is folded to form a makeshift pillow under my head. This posture begins my practice. Its effect is a delicate balance that opens and lifts my chest, while also lengthening the back of my neck. It is designed to allow my breath to enter my chest and torso more freely.

The bustle of life has begun around me. I hear the bathroom door latch and water pour from the faucet. In these last few yogic breaths, I can feel that my diaphragm is slightly gripped—it is the anticipation of contact with others. I sink inward and feel presence in the backs of my heels. The effect is a softening of my diaphragm.

I marvel with a thought. After all that I have been through, the ability to connect awareness through my heels represents one of my greatest accomplishments—something so subtle, something that seems so ordinary. I am not walking, nor do I feel courageous, but I have worked hard for such a moment. It has taken patience, persistence, and a willingness to feel vulnerable. It has taken a different kind of strength.

I hear the sound of feet tramping down the hallway. I feel Paul peering down at me. "Why are you sleeping on the floor, Papa?" As I slowly open my eyes, I am already smiling.

2

My Body Broken

The year was 1978. After three and a half days, I simply opened my eyes. As I met my brother's frantic gaze, relief lit across his face. He squeezed my hand, quietly slipped out of the room, and returned a few seconds later with our mother.

My waking had occurred slowly. First, I moved from the silence and into a dream. I remember hearing noises: a heart monitor, a respirator, various beeps—the sounds of lifesaving technology. My thirteen-year-old reaction, "Wow, a realistic dream . . . like on TV . . . cool." My endurance spent, I drifted back into silence. Other times, I was roused by hushed voices, edged with seriousness, but they too were fleeting, certainly nothing adequate to lift my slumber.

But then the dream became frightening. While again admiring its realism, I began to notice a connection between one of the sounds and my own breathing. Sleepily, I attempted to separate them. *Okay, next time I hear the sound, I'll hold my breath. Ready . . .* My chest jerked and inflated without me. *Maybe I wasn't ready. Try again . . .* Same result. Something was out of my control. As a child who had suffered from horrible nightmares, I had learned how to exit unwanted dreams, and I wanted out of this one. I moved outward toward waking but to no avail. My chest continued to heave without my consent.

This scene played over and over. I would become vaguely aware of certain sounds, try to hold my breath, fail, and then float back into the comforting silence—that place just below sleep, which renders action unnecessary. Over time, though, my efforts became a source of panic. I fought to win, to make what was happening a dream. But the more I failed, the more frightened I became, and in turn the harder I fought. My resistance became a problem, so much so that my doctors were forced to medicate me. Without knowing it, I had begun to fight against the respirator, the very machine that was keeping me alive. But still I admire that young boy who struggled to wake from a dream by reclaiming his own breath. He could have gone back to seventh grade, back to playing on three basketball teams, and made a vow not to watch so much television. Instead, he woke up to quite another life.

"Matt, you gotta make it . . . you gotta pull through . . . I don't know if I can go on without you." With my brother's imploring voice, I began to consciously realize that something was very wrong. His words rang through my head as a continuous plea, a relentless invasion of my sleep, though in reality, this wasn't the case. Intensive care visits were restricted to ten minutes every hour, so he couldn't have been there that much. Still, for me, his words were a mantra, a guiding beacon leading me through the silence and back into that room. Somehow, I traveled to the sound of his voice.

Once my eyes adjusted, my mother's face irreparably broke my protective silence. On the left side, from the corner of her eye to the side of her jaw, was a gruesome bruise—black, muted with purple, yellow, and gray. At that moment, waking life snapped into focus. Up until then, I had remained an observer. My lifeless presence had yet to do anything, had yet to commit me to anything. I was merely a body-ghost. But as the helpless pain in my mother's eyes washed through the body I could not feel, the first outward signs of living trickled down my cheeks. Something terrible had happened to my family.

My gaze traveled between their faces, between my mother and brother, between Paula and James. My mother looked pale. Below her curly, strawberry blonde hair, her eyes had always carried a touch of sadness, as if anticipating great suffering. Now that sadness was realized. My brother's sharp chin and long eyelashes were softened by a mop of dishwater blond hair. Seventeen years had brought him the look of the man before the man, that off-balance, in-between vigor that someday would transform into stabilizing strength. Emanating from both of them, I felt a loving, desperate emptiness.

The room's only rhythm was the respirator's uneven bursts and the synchronous heaving of my chest. Silence lingered between us. Within it hung, just for an instant, images of our previous lives—canoe trips, dinner-table discussions, laughter, long car rides—images of a family now slipping away. But in that moment, just before the present wrenched from us an unconditional surrender, a truth coursed through me—*my family needed me to live*. I would accept whatever was coming. I knew I had to show them

that I was going to be okay, that I would join them in this painfully uncertain future. All this happened before we shared words.

I tried to speak but could not. When I motioned for a pen and
paper, a surprising relief crossed their faces. I had been knocked
out, so there had been no way to know the extent of my injuries,
and especially if there had been brain damage. My mother and
brother had lived with this unknown for three and a half days. At
least that concern ended as I wrote *Dad and Laura?* My mother
slowly closed her eyes; my brother looked up to the ceiling.

"They didn't make it," my brother choked. *My father and
sister dead?* Unable to gulp or cry out . . . into the silence my new
life went.

My next scrawl: *What happened?*

My brother's cracking voice: "We were in a car accident . . .
skidded off a bridge."

You two?

"I jammed my shoulder and mom hit her head pretty hard, but
we're fine."

Where are we?

"Mercy Hospital in Des Moines, Iowa."

Me? There was a long pause as they looked at each other. When
my brother turned back to me, I saw tears flooding his eyes.

"You got pretty banged up."

My mom broke in, "Matt, you've been in a coma. It's serious."

I can't feel my legs.

"You've broken your back. They think you're paralyzed." Time
stood still. Disconnected images of walking moved through my
mind and into the darkness. "They say you'll never walk again."

I felt numb. The death of my father and sister hardly registered—I took it in as a piece of information, like a report of the day's weather. Instead, I stayed locked on the feeling that my remaining family needed me to live. I'd like to say there was something heroic in this stance, but there wasn't. I did not grasp the threat to my continued existence and then rally to beat the odds. Nothing was that conscious, nothing that willful. The invisible strength came from somewhere much deeper. Survival took charge without my choosing.

My focus also intuitively shifted away from the decimated state of my body. I could not dwell on the extent of my physical damage. In addition to crushing my upper thoracic vertebrae at T4–6, I had broken my neck at the very top—the atlas vertebra—the one that literally holds up the head and protects primary life functions, including breathing. I had also broken both my wrists, filled a lung with fluid, and sustained an internal injury to my pancreas. This last problem knocked my digestive system off-line for what turned out to be months.

My injuries were beyond my comprehension. I could sense, however, that they threatened more than my physical body. My psyche, my sense of living was also under attack. I was enveloped by a feeling of death. My body was without its own breath, a powerful pointing toward an immediate end. Moreover, through the acute absence of my father and sister, the imprint of death surrounded my bed, so much so that even to this day my mother, brother, and I cannot dismiss the viability of ghosts. Finally, my mother's and brother's expressions poured forth the sallow hue of tears, grief, and devastating loss—death as it is absorbed by the living.

I could not control what was going to happen, but I could control how I perceived my situation. I needed to find a path, a way to keep focused on going forward. So I told myself a story, a healing story: *My mother and brother desperately need me to live.* It was like whistling in the dark—a way to feel rhythm despite being engulfed in the unknown. This healing story guided my tenuous sense of living through disastrous waters, an unconscious move wrought by the brilliance of survival.

～

During the fleeting moments in intensive care when I did feel connected to my body, *wow* did it hurt. Often, just being rolled from side to side was enough to knock me unconscious. I was in a state beyond my comprehension—too many things were going on, going wrong. My sense of feeling overwhelmed was only heightened by my inability to speak and connect directly with others. I spent five days in Mercy Hospital doing the only things I could—lying flat and listening. Whether I was in a coma or awake, people around me spoke as they saw fit.

Over time, my brother told me the story of what had happened. I remember none of it—not the accident or any of the day it occurred. I don't even remember the last meal I ate with my whole family. In fact, I have only sketchy memories of the preceding weekend. My brother has been my witness.

Ever since I can remember, my family had spent Thanksgiving

with my mom's sister, Aunt Kathy, and her family. This entailed two long, straight-shot drives on I-35 between Duluth, Minnesota, and Kansas City, Missouri. The main constant on these trips was Iowa corn. That year we did even more driving because we detoured to pick up my sister, who was in her junior year at the University of Iowa in Iowa City. The five of us piled into a car built for four and spent cramped, chaotic, but lovely time together as only families can. There were candy wrappers and comic books and gum, games of hangman and packed sandwiches and sleep. All too quickly, Thanksgiving weekend was over and it was time for the long drive home.

This was a dreary Sunday, overcast and slightly misting. We left a little before eight in the morning. About an hour into the drive, we stopped for gas. Apparently, I bought some gum that came with a superball. (I know this because my brother kept the ball in his pocket throughout my hospital stay.) The five of us packed ourselves back into the car. My father was driving. My brother, having recently gone past six feet tall, had finagled his way into the front passenger seat because he needed extra legroom. I sat in the back seat behind my father. My sister sat in the middle, and our mother sat behind my brother. None of us back-seat passengers wore seat belts. In 1978, the "buckle up" media blitz had yet to occur. The temperature outside was near freezing. Although a snowstorm was forecast for later, it seemed like a harmless day to travel.

As we approached an overpass just across the Iowa border from Missouri, my father pulled into the left lane to pass another vehicle. Once past the car, we hit a patch of ice—quite a surprise, considering it was only misting. We skidded to the right; my father corrected. Suddenly we hit a dry patch of road, and because the wheel was turned hard left, the car shot sharply in that direction. Our left front wheel got caught over the road's edge, causing our car to tumble down the embankment. We rolled three times, front to back.

My brother came awake to the flat rhythm of windshield wipers. He saw that my father sat dead, belted in his seat, his head crushed through the side window by the force of impact. He could hear our mother moving behind him, but my sister and I were nowhere to be seen. He forced his door open and stumbled around the site. Off to the left of the car, he found my sister lying in some tall grass. One look, and he knew she wasn't going to make it. Her neck was horribly broken, her head impossibly crooked over her left shoulder, her futile gasping for breath obviously short-lived. Still, there was no me. My brother frantically trampled through the grass. Panicked, he fell silent. Imperceptibly at first, then louder and louder, he detected a guttural noise back near the car. As he rushed to the sound, he clearly heard moaning and groaning, and a long run of choice cussing. He told me, "When I heard you swearing to beat the band, I knew you were okay." He found my body right beside the tilting car, wedged almost underneath it. He saw that I, too, was struggling for breath. He ran up the embankment, flagged down a car, secured help. He then fainted near the scene.

Amazingly, he had flagged down a nurse and a paramedic, athough there was little they could do. My brother awoke a few moments later to confirmation of what he already knew. There was no hope for our father or for our sister. Although things looked bad for me, I was still alive, so there was a chance. The wait, the wait, the wait. An ambulance had been called, but it had to travel more than thirty miles and took nearly a half-hour to arrive. After saying good-bye to her husband and her only daughter, my mom wandered around aimlessly, gathering up the clothing and personal belongings spewed by the violence. Already she was starting to pick up the pieces. There was no rhyme nor reason to what she was doing. My brother, on the other hand, sat next to me, praying.

I was turning blue by the time the ambulance appeared. The blue continued to deepen as we approached the county hospital in Leon, Iowa. I needed that respirator; I needed its unnatural rhythm. My time in Leon was short, a little over twenty-four hours.

The nature of my injuries was somewhat mysterious. At first, there was some hope that I might just wake up and be relatively fine. As I continued to slumber, however, the concern increased proportionally. Obviously something had happened to my ability to breathe, but what? I had no apparent cuts or bruises, and yet my upper thoracic region must have been hammered. My heart was the initial concern. My condition was so critical that nothing could be done but watch, wait, and hope that I might weather the storm. The doctor stayed with me through the night. It wasn't until the next morning that Dr. Sullivan began to suspect an additional injury. He responded to my mom's questioning eyes.

"For what Matt's been through, he's doing just fine. The worst is over. I think he's going to pull through." He paused. "But something else worries me. The whole night I was with him,

Matt never moved his legs. That's not a good sign. I'm sending him for x-rays, but I suspect a spinal cord injury."

"No . . . how could you have . . . ?"

"Missed it? I don't know . . . he arrived in such critical condition that I could barely keep up with keeping him alive. I can't believe I didn't catch it earlier. I'm so sorry."

"Will he be paralyzed?"

"It's too soon to be sure. We'll know more after the x-rays . . . but it looks as if he already is."

The spinal cord injury, coupled with the fracture at the top of my neck, put my case beyond the reach of the county hospital. Although my condition was still critical, and moving me posed a mortal risk, Dr. Sullivan immediately arranged for my transport to Des Moines. The hope was to get me better care. Unfortunately, that turned out not to be the case.

So began the five-day, behind-the-scenes saga at Mercy Hospital. The waiting room outside the ICU had no windows. The trembling fluorescent lights could muster only an unnatural dimness. Colors lost contrast; reading was nearly impossible, and focus was gained solely by rubbing one's eyes. The room's only intended reprieve—a poorly done mural—covered the entire wall directly across from the stark and uncomfortable chairs. Its subject was a dark and ominous wooded scene traveling up a distant hill. Its effect was to enhance the room's surreal character. My mother and brother struggled for equilibrium.

Worse, the doctors literally avoided them. The orthopedist and the neurologist made their rounds at five in the morning, making no effort to be available for consultation. So my family waited,

waited for something to change, for me to open my eyes, for time to move forward. They were told nothing about my prognosis, about potential treatment or strategy. When I finally awoke, there was still no contact from the doctors. At five the next morning, my mom tracked down one of the attending physicians. He wouldn't say much but agreed to set up a meeting with the neurologist for the next day.

In the meantime, my favorite nurse, Marilyn, approached my mom.

"Mrs. Sanford, I shouldn't be telling you this, but you need to get Matt out of here." She looked my mom straight in the eyes. "The care he's getting . . . it's not good enough. His injuries are too severe . . . the doctors don't know what they're doing. We're turning him from side to side, and he's only wearing a soft collar brace. His neck is broken, for god's sake. It's dangerous . . . it's wrong."

"We have a meeting with them today."

"I know, but I've talked to some of the other nurses, and we all agree: No matter what they tell you, get Matt out of here. If he's going to survive, he needs more-aggressive treatment. It can't wait any longer."

"What should I do?"

"Demand his release and get him to another hospital. They may tell you that he might not survive the trip. But I can tell you one thing for sure . . . he won't survive if he stays here."

Mutiny among the caregivers. My mother went to the meeting as planned, hoping that Marilyn was overreacting, hoping that it wasn't true. The neurologist was an older man, his body tired, his hair completely gray. He was obviously from the "old school" and nearing the end of his career. At first, the meeting was typical of one with a doctor—confusing and evasive. My mom finally brought it to a head.

"Why aren't we doing more? Why aren't we doing something to protect Matt's neck?" Standing firm, she feigned authority.

"Your son's condition is far from stable. We can't do anything without the risk of making things worse. As far as his neck goes, that's not his most pressing problem."

"What are you saying?"

"Look, your son has suffered catastrophic injuries. There isn't one thing we can definitely do to make things better. His case presents a myriad of issues. Although he's now awake, he can't breathe on his own. His heart appears to be okay, but it's not functioning as we would like. There must be some internal injury, because everything in his digestive system has stopped working. Who knows if and when that will ever reverse itself. I've never seen anything like this. Quite frankly, his broken bones are not his worst problem. Even if he makes it through this initial crisis, it only gets worse. His spinal cord injury will never go away. It presents complications you don't even want to imagine right now."

"So basically, you're waiting to see if he might die?"

"Sometimes it's better to let your loved one go."

"His name is Matt, and we're not waiting for him to die," my mom said, stepping forward. "We want him discharged . . . we're going someplace else."

"I'm sorry. I can't do that. As a doctor, I cannot take an action that will make my patient's condition worse. Your son will die if he is moved."

Immediately, my mom contacted my sister's godfather, an orthopedic surgeon. He made the arrangements for my transfer to the Mayo Clinic in Rochester, Minnesota. Then she called my father's law partner. "Get Matt the hell out of this hospital. They won't release him!" Bruce drove down from Duluth that afternoon. He made one phone call to the neurologist and said simply, "We won't sue you if you agree immediately to . . ." That was that. He then contacted an ambulance service that had a mobile home vehicle that doubled as an intensive care unit. I was off to the Mayo Clinic the next day.

I remember being taken down the hallway—respirator, at least three IVs, a heart monitor, and who knows what else in tow—toward this huge ambulance. Out of nowhere, a man wearing a big silver belt buckle yelled "Hold it!" and stopped us right on the spot. "You're telling me that this boy has a broken neck, and no one is holding it steady! Who the hell is in charge here? Scratch that! Whoever it is, you're done. I'm taking over." This belt buckle was a nurse-practitioner, the person in charge of my care during transport. Finally, something was happening.

According to my mom, it was a tense five-and-a-half-hour drive through some hideous weather. I wouldn't know; I was drugged and out of it. My head was held, positioned to look straight up at the ceiling, the entire time. Eventually, after radio consultation with the doctors at the Mayo Clinic, I was taken off the respirator. For the first time in more than five days, I was my own rhythm-maker, my own connection to time. Although the fresh air pouring through my body was shockingly cold, it was there with my consent.

3

Out of Body

$Aggressive$ treatment was what we wanted, aggressive treatment is what we got. I am met by a team of doctors and brought into an open area. There is no time lapse; there is only action. A curtain is drawn and suddenly I am enclosed in an artificial room. I suspect this is an emergency room, but there's no telling. The view is not great from flat on my back.

The lights overhead are bright and hot, and yet my vision is dim. The faces and voices are like shadows, conversations swirling, no apparent direction. I am surrounded by many bodies. Two men are standing particularly close, by each of my shoulders. They whisper to each other right over my chest. The quality of their voices reveals their importance: crisp, authoritative, calm, with a confident edge. But they have no faces. I see only their arms, hands, torsos, and the underside of their chins. They are holding some sort of hand tools. Unknown to me, I am about to have four metal screws twisted directly into my skull. It is the first step in getting a halo cast, the ultimate in neck stabilization.

Suddenly, two other men appear from above me and hold down my arms. Two screwdrivers move toward my temples. My skin breaks, warmness runs into my hair. The pain is sharp and getting sharper. A horrible sound explodes in my head, not from the outside in, but from the inside out. The screws continue to twist into my skull. The pressure is slow at first, building, and then exponential. My head no longer exists in three dimensions, no space between collapsing sides, just two rocks grinding each other.

Suddenly, it's done. A semblance of vision returns. Then, out of nowhere, it begins again . . . twisting right above each ear. This time, I am not in that body; there is no subject of that experience. I land in profound silence, watching a boy. He is on a table, a sheet is draped loosely over his lower body. He seems so small. Time is off-track, and I am everywhere. The doctors move, but things are held up, stretched out, turned over, pulled apart—a silent movie on a faltering projector. Suddenly, time finds its rhythm, sounds appear again, the vacuum is broken. A timid voice that I recognize as my own, "Somebody help me."

A path of realization—big or small—almost always starts bumpy. In my case, I was thrown off a cliff. In retrospect, I realize that this halo experience altered the course of my life. It left me with an insight. At a moment of intense physical pain, the fragile state of my living was able to "move away" from my body. The potential for dislocation between mind and body was dramatically revealed. The insight, however, was not the ability to disassociate. It was the silence that I experienced while it happened. This silence not only allowed me to separate from my body, but it was also sticky enough to maintain a life-preserving connection. Somehow I stayed connected to that boy below me. The silence within my consciousness both separated me and connected me simultaneously. This paradoxical insight still guides my life.

⤶

When I wake from my halo cast experience, I am in a different room. My awareness is scattered; it comes in phases, sometimes almost crisp, other times threadbare. Somehow, I hear the date— December second. Tomorrow is my mother's birthday, and I need to show her, show everyone, that I am holding on, that I am okay. With my recently reacquired voice, I ask for my Aunt Kathy. Weakly, I inform her of my mom's impending birthday. "Will you please get her something for me? She needs something." There is a pause. I am on my back, and my neck is in traction. It's impossible to turn my head. I push my eyes hard left. Silent tears are running down her cheeks, "Are you sure?" Yes, I say. She buys a silk scarf, green and tan, in a design I can hardly register. It is surprisingly nice for a hospital gift shop. I am pleased.

It seems like I see this scarf every day for weeks. My mother wears it rolled up and clasped around her neck, with a tan turtleneck sweater and slacks. Truthfully, I have no idea how often she wears it. The hours, the days, even the minutes have dropped their focus. But for me, the scarf is imprinted on my mind, a beacon of my choice.

Although getting a present for my mother felt noble and necessary, it was motivated by denial. For the six days since the accident, my mother and brother poured everything imaginable—love, prayers, hope, fear, desperation, and, most powerfully, imprints of themselves—into my fragile state of living. They needed to tip the balance toward living: Three of five surviving was manageable; but if three of five die, the dam breaks, and death overwhelms our family. They gave as only loved ones can, throwing lifelines into a seamless dark. Finally, I reached a place where I could grab the other end. I pulled hard and fast. I didn't want to feel my body. I wanted to feel my family instead.

I am spitting into a metallic, crescent-shaped bowl. My saliva hangs and drops like a gummy paste, its cotton whiteness plopping against the shiny gray. The bowl's design is intended to encircle the neck below the chin and allows for mess-free spitting. These mouth commodes are standard issue in a hospital and provide bedridden patients with a place to spit such things as toothpaste and mouthwash. Simple cleanliness habits like brushing my teeth, gargling with mouthwash, even picking my nose are beyond my reach. My arms are too weak, and I am lying on a Foster frame in the children's intensive care unit at the Mayo Clinic.

A Foster frame is hard for me to describe because I have never actually seen one. I have only been on one. They are used in critical care situations for maximal stabilization of back and neck injuries. I will live on one for weeks. The structure itself is made of two canvas stretchers attached to a frame; the frame allows the stretchers to turn 180 degrees abruptly. Every two hours I am sandwiched between the stretchers—one has an opening for my face—and in a whirl of motion my body can still feel but my mind cannot fathom, I am turned from stomach to back or from back to stomach.

When on my stomach—my face protruding through the circular hole—the metallic mouth commode positioned about two feet below is a godsend. I have a tube running through my nose, down my throat, and into my stomach. A constant stream of greenish-black juices flows through this plumbing. It is spillage from my distraught digestive system, one that has lost any order in its functioning. My body is pouring its highly effective but corrosive digestive juices into all the wrong places. Thus far, they have burned a hole in my stomach and given me a screaming case of heartburn. My center chest is on fire. And the smell—oh how these juices smell. I now intimately grasp the guttural source of the word *bile*. The tube itself has given me a raging sore throat. My saliva must not take the road to my stomach. So I spit and spit, but I don't really spit. I drop, it drops, into the bowl—*plink, plink, plink*—rhythmically marking time. And time passes, slowly, very slowly.

While I am in this state, my mother reads to me. I can hardly hear, but it doesn't matter. The cadence of her words holds me steady. The grayness of my sensation tells me that I am not really in that body, the one strewn over that Foster frame. I am above, not looking, just hovering—a presence spread thin, very thin. I am thankful for the sound of my mother's voice, the reading of words, the turning of pages, and the occasional question. Blindly, I stay in that room and time continues to pass.

More than twenty-five years later, I still carry that feeling of floating in grayness above the Foster frame. I know now that it is a perceptual expression of the silence, a dullness created by the separation of mind and body. It is also the sensation produced when the energies of life and death are overtly mixed. This is one of the mixtures that the practice of yoga seeks to clarify.

It is easy to see how yoga clarifies the connection between mind and body. The mindful practice of particular physical movements combines mind and body into a unified experience. Take one part away, however—for example, the full attention of the mind—and the overall experience changes significantly. The yoga practitioner becomes increasingly aware of the vital role that both mind and body play in any action.

Harder to imagine is how yoga can also clarify our sense of life and death. Both life and death exist within the potential of the mind-body relationship—death being the complete absence of a connection between the two, and life being dependent on some degree of connection. In yoga, as one explores the fluctuating relationship between mind and body, one gains glimpses into the continuum of living and dying.

One day I notice that I am next to a window. There is talk about an almost constant stream of geese passing by the opening. This migration is a renowned seasonal event—masses of fowl flee-

ing the snapping cold of the Canadian winter to find warm, nourishing waters much farther south. Their major flight pattern
covers the airspace over Rochester, Minnesota, and the sightline
out my window. I cannot see them though, and my brother begins
to problem-solve. He buys a tabletop facial mirror that rotates and
carefully positions it so I can see the geese flying by.

Arrow after arrow, these geese formations pass the window
like silent waves. For me, their flow is continuous, for time has
lost its edges. Most arrows are perfectly symmetrical, as if formed
in some kind of mold. Occasionally, they are skewed, so that a
contingent of three or four fly a little off center, a little behind.
The unity of the arrow is not compromised, however, only mis-
shapen, like the subtle differences among similar rocks. Once in a
while, there is a goose that doesn't fit with the arrow and flies a
good distance behind. I wonder if it chooses this place, chooses to
fly outside of the group. Perhaps it fell out of position and will
soon reclaim its spot. Or maybe it's losing the connection between
it and the group. Maybe it doesn't matter. Silence.

When I tire of the geese, my brother finds a balancing marvel
in the gift shop. On one side a silver ball rests in opposition to a
silver seagull on the other. Exactly in the middle, a small sharp
pin rests in a stand; the whole thing sits on the floor below me.
The result is a delicate balance between the ball and the bird,
making the arm holding the two capable of circular movement.
Although I cannot set it in motion myself, others can. I watch for
countless hours and am grateful for a way to mark time.

In a couple of weeks, I will be moved to a room with a television in the upper corner. My brother finds another mirror. He

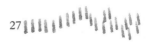

perfectly positions the mirrors so that the TV's image is reflected twice before it meets my eyes. Now I look forward to 3:30, when Spiderman begins. For a thirteen-year-old boy, this is progress.

⌒

The car accident did not happen to one person, not even to one family. It happened to a group, to a circle of connection, to a community. We move forward into uncharted territory together.

The core of my support is comprised of my mother; my brother; my Aunt Kathy; my father's best friend, Lauren; and my sister's almost-fiancé, Bob. Bob will be around a lot during my stay in Rochester. I do not realize how amazing this is until much later. We had heard his name for about two years and met him once when he was brought home to meet the family. We all suspected that he might be added to our ranks through marriage, but we didn't know for sure. But he chooses to be here now, bonding quickly as a brother and a virtual son to my mother. Of course, he is here to support, but his presence also softens the grief, both his and ours. For me, my sister is still twenty and not exactly dead yet. I watch her through the sadness in Bob's eyes.

These people hand me off quietly, as if deftly passing a baton. One visitor is reading to me, an extra chair is pulled up, a book handed off, a shared odd encounter, a quick burst of laughter, and one becomes two. Another arrives, now briefly three, two leave for lunch, back to one, a new reading voice emerges, and I am in contact the whole time. So skillful are these exchanges, I never feel awkward or needy. I feel part of a group, of a team, but with the perpetual permission to drift off. There are no awkward silences, no forced interactions, nothing is wasted, just shared spaces—silent sustenance among the waiting.

And yet this group also lives outside my room. They stand together in the cafeteria line and survey tired food propped up by heat lamps. They contemplate Jell-O with fruit in it, brown lettuce, rubber tomatoes, Salisbury steak, scary-looking gravy, and instant mashed potatoes. They walk down poorly lit hallways, past lime-green walls, whimpering voices, through countless double doors, and to the drone of unrelenting televisions. All this just to find an outside door, to feel the natural warmth of sunlight, or to have a fresh hit of uncirculated air. Somehow they find enough nourishment and bring it back to me, always me, carrying me forward. We are a rotating team as the timeless gray of trauma threatens to swallow us.

But the world has not suddenly stopped. My seventh-grade classes continue without me. The varsity basketball team continues its undefeated season without me on the bench. Jobs continue, cars idle, people shovel snow, have dinner, and sleep in their own beds. So too the call of normal living pulls at my people. Lauren must return to his engineering and architecture firm. My Aunt Kathy has her own family and her own job coordinating the remedial reading program in the Kansas City public schools. They leave amid silence, tearful laughter, and promises of return. I feel them depart, feel the force of what has happened as the dance hall begins to clear. Bob must return to the University of Minnesota.

meanwhile, the world goes on

angela

29

He is studying business administration. I will see him often on weekends.

My mother decides to hold fort in Rochester until she can personally bring me back to Duluth. But my brother . . . my brother must return home, an advance scout into an empty and unrecognizable life. He is in the midst of his senior year, his banner year of high school. He is tied as the top-ranked student in his class; he is the elected treasurer of the student forum; and he is a multisport athlete. All this and a wonderful girlfriend await him back in "normal" time. But how? Mid-December in Duluth is not particularly encouraging. The leaves are gone, the grass is brown. Lake Superior wind rips through your clothes, and the cold, sharp air alerts your nose that a long, dark winter lies ahead. Life stripped naked, barren, and waiting.

How does he return to the death of our previous life? I cannot fathom what he is experiencing. I can only feel that he is leaving, and I am scared. The world makes more sense around my older brother; he sets things right. But now he steps through a time-warp and into his own private silence. I cannot help him. I can only long for his return.

He survives the winter of his senior year, alone, in an empty house, cooking his own meals, and with four-fifths of his family in other worlds. I insist that he come every weekend, every bit of Christmas vacation. He makes the five-hour drive from Duluth to Rochester through the tundra of Minnesota winter. I do not know what I ask of him, nor how he gives it. I just know that I need him. He will graduate at the top of his class, having lettered

in baseball, his eyes vacant but determined. He is the unseen hero.
I love him.

Thankfully, more people appear, other reservoirs of strength.
My mom rents a two-bedroom motel suite, equipped with a kitch-
enette. They come to stay with her and visit me. My mom's female
peers are the best company. They expect little, accept much, and
give tons. They share meals with my mom and talk to her late at
night when the ache of silence is most acute. And they read to me,
giving my mother a break, giving her time to absorb or just feel
numb. The best are Lauren's wife Catharine, my mom's friend
Ann, and our cousin Joan. They spend time with me, just willing
to sit, be quiet as I spit, not wince when I beg for another pain
shot. Always willing to extend maternal love to a hurting child.

Other visitors are not so easy. They drive a long way and feel
that they must accomplish something, achieve a definite interaction. I do not have interaction to give, but I find myself taking
care of these visitors. Little things exhaust me: three consecutive
replies, traveling with them through old memories, and, especially, knowing that I am not really there.

Eventually, I see my two best friends. Mark Drexler lives across
a shared driveway. His dad, Dr. Drexler, makes the drive to
Rochester so we can connect. I can't say that I am excited; I'm not

anything, really, except vaguely scared. Seeing my friend makes my experience more real, makes me feel what I am and what he is not. Mark struts in and gulps; his dad stands awkwardly behind him. I am tired and have very little to give. I fall in and out of time; there are long pauses where I drift. I smell of death. It becomes time for me to be turned, and they must step out. Because the drawn curtain makes only an artificial room, I hear frightened sobs and Mark saying, "He's going to die, isn't he!?" Apparently, I don't look so good.

This fact is confirmed with Roger's visit. Roger and I have been friends since we were three. During that year, we had our first and only full-fledged fight. It was in the neighbor's yard, over the use of a tree stump. I drew first tears, but then he knocked my head into the disputed real estate. We sat there, looking at each other, both crying tears of shock and betrayal. That day we entered into a silent pact: Fighting with each other was simply too painful and not to be done again.

When Roger comes around the curtain, his face goes a greener shade of pale. He tries conversation but stumbles; and, thirty seconds after arriving, he faints and plummets toward the floor. Upon reviving, the visit starts for real. It is a good visit. I am told that Roger has the flu, but the source of his drop through the silence is clear.

4

Which Family Were We?

The car accident happened to my family: to my father, my mother, my sister, my brother, and me. It also happened to Loren, Paula, Laura, James, and Matthew. They were and are individuals, each with voice intonations, unique ways of walking, different laughs, and distinct destinies. We made up a family, and we all crashed down that embankment together.

My father, Loren, was an attorney, a partner in a leading firm in Duluth, Minnesota. He was born during the Depression, the second son of farmers who barely eked out a living on 164 acres of average farmland. He grew up poor, with the year-to-year uncertainty that comes with farm life. He was the first to leave the family farm, going to college and law school at the University of Minnesota and then choosing a life away from his heritage by marrying a big-city girl.

Loren was a bright man, at times quite stoic, and dead at the age of forty-seven. He was thoughtful and powerful and loved to argue. He loved to take any opposing position, no matter how outrageous, and carry it to the breaking point. For example, he was a delegate to the Republican National Convention during the 1968 presidential campaign. He went down to Miami, wearing black horn-rimmed glasses and a green plaid sports coat, all under the auspices of supporting Richard Nixon, and then promptly voted for Nelson Rockefeller. This fateful whim so outraged the Minnesota Republican caucus that he was quietly but firmly purged from the party.

Loren was athletic without being a great athlete, physically strong without an imposing presence. Being color-blind, he was a frightful dresser. Nowhere worse than on the golf course—imagine bright purple shorts, black socks, and a brown shirt. Unless my mother was around to stop him, he would ignore the entreaties of his embarrassed kids. This was particularly painful for my brother and me, as we often caddied for him. I could never tell if he wore such attire because he was color-blind or just loved to push our buttons.

Wherever his life brought him, my father, at core, remained a farmer at heart: deeply connected to the land, to the discipline of hard work, and to planning for the future—all the while longing for the outdoors.

My mother, Paula, was also born during the Depression but to a family of city dwellers. Her father was a charming man, an attorney, and a generally tame alcoholic. Her mother was an amazingly bright woman, was well-read, possessed an unfaltering memory, but was quietly broken by the addictive habits of her husband. Early on, Paula learned to willfully see the world as normal, despite the peaks and valleys of living with an alcoholic. She took care of things, exuded a quiet confidence, and made things all right for her younger sister. To this day, my mother's most powerful quality is how deeply she loves—sometimes staying behind the scenes, sometimes invisible, always loyal, and always willing to see the best in people. She is kind and graceful and deeply committed to the well-being of her loved ones.

Paula is also an artist, primarily a painter. In addition to making a wonderful and stable home for her family, she has always found time to create: taking the world—beautiful as she sees it—and translating its designs and patterns to paper and canvas. Imagine her in our damp basement—no windows and the lights overhead are quite dim. On a cheap plastic table sits the "Orange Peeler," a ninety-dollar phonograph with an orange plastic lid and orange-faced speakers. The year is 1970. The music is either Judy Collins or Joni Mitchell, depending on how the six albums are stacked on the record player. I am with her, too young for school, and playing under a card table. My secret house is covered with a quilt, securing the hidden surveillance I need for playing spy. My mother is wearing an old pair of slacks, and an oversized man's dress shirt drapes her body. Her hair is held at bay by a folded scarf, worn as a headband. Long pauses ensue as she tilts her head, rocks from foot to foot, and absorbs her work through the pores of her skin. As she extends her sense of beauty outward, I hear her paintbrush clinking out of the coffee cup, swishing through the cleansing water, mixing colors, and then rubbing against the textured surface of the canvas.

This scene is repeated again and again over a lifetime, both with and without my presence—when I am there, when I am at school, before I was born, and after I move away for college. Having produced literally hundreds of pieces, she leaves quite a legacy for a woman who walks so lightly on her feet, sets things down so gently, and softly hums to herself as she paints.

My sister, Laura, seven and a half years my elder, announced to our mom, "There is no need for any more babysitters." This when she was nine. Laura was like a second mother and sister wrapped into one, intuitive enough to recognize changes in me and shift our relationship accordingly. For my eighth birthday, she gave me an oversized navy blue jersey, inscribed—in fire red—with SANFORD and the number 8. Earlier that year, she had joined an intramural touch-football team and received her own jersey. She saw how taken I was with it and with the idea of being on a team. So she made me my own team. For my ninth birthday, she took me out to breakfast before school. Having recently received her driver's license, she took me to a Perkins restaurant—just the two of us—and then drove us around with the radio blaring. She showed me places where the high school kids hung out—Seven Bridges Road and Hawk's Ridge—granting me precious glimpses into her older life. For my tenth birthday, she gave me my first rock and roll album: The Doobie Brothers, *Living on the Fault Line*. With this gift, she sent me into a new world of music, and I learned every word in every song.

Laura was five foot six with brownish-blonde hair and was beautifully left-handed. Her penmanship was exquisite, not because it followed prescribed rules but because of the feeling it conveyed: precise, perfectly slanted, but flowing—fat, round a's and p's; unabashed loops around g's, f's, and y's; and perfectly round o's. Her writing looked so alive.

She is lying in bed, knees propped in the air, and using her lap as a table. She is in high school. I watch, wondering what she writes, wondering how she stays quiet for so long. If I say anything, I become an annoying little brother and no longer welcome. So I admire the discipline of her journal writing, happy just to feel the outline of her intent. Her hands are soft but strong, her long fingers firmly clasping an extra-thick ballpoint pen. As her left hand slides smoothly across the page, a smile breaks cleanly through her expression. Even now, some twenty-five years later, as I survey one of these diaries, I know better than to read the particular words. They are hers. I must simply love the feel of her handwriting.

When she died, Laura was twenty—just coming into her own. She had transformed from an average-looking and slightly overweight girl to a sexy and beautiful woman. An understated yet powerful confidence became her most attractive feature. This was not always the case. She had ample friends in high school but was by no means popular. The result was that she tried to see beyond her age, to be quietly above the fray. She worked to become wise.

Laura liked making beautiful things, wrote poetry, and read avidly. She was the best storyteller I have ever known. In her short life, Laura was able to transform her natural tendency to give to others into a source of creativity. This was the Laura who took care of me when I was young, who listened to my life, saw it, smiled, and returned it to me. This was the Laura who awakened in college to major in art, her creativity finding a formal, artistic expression. Seeing and making designs was what she did best. She finally realized that being an artist could be her own path and not just an imitation of her mother's.

But still, her greatest strength was her power of perception. So thoughtful, so aware of other people's feelings—qualities she exhibited without drawing attention to herself. She simply perceived, making you feel—in your bones—that she saw what was invisible about you. Her gifts of perception were powerful because they affirmed the secrets of who you were. She was easily loved.

My brother, James, and I have always shared friends, even before the accident. This is somewhat surprising, considering that he is four and a half years my elder. Hero worship of an older brother is common, but James handled mine so gracefully. I wanted to do everything he did, and he was patiently obliging. He was the best source of entertainment I had growing up, making gripping games out of everything—and nothing. Twist hockey, a dignified precursor to video games, wasn't just a contest between the Boston Bruins and the New York Rangers. It was the Stanley Cup, and we knew the names of all the best players and played our own best-of-seven series.

Our backyard was the neighborhood Wiffle-ball park. Our green-shingled roof was called the "Green Monster" after the legendary fence at Fenway Park. A rotted, cut-to-the-ground tree stump was first base, the lilac bush was second, a select branch of the gigantic red pine was third, and a natural mound was home plate. A ball hit over the house was a home run, one hit down the driveway was a ground rule double, as was a ball lost in my mom's garden. But it didn't stop there. We kept replaying the 1973 World Series between the Oakland Athletics and the New York Mets.

Since my brother and I were the best pitchers—we could throw the best junk—we were always on opposing teams. He was Ken Holtzman, the brash young pitcher for the A's, and I was John Matlock, a crafty veteran from the Mets and my adopted namesake. It never grew tiresome.

My brother convinced the neighborhood rug rats to assume roles. This was true whether we were playing Wiffle ball, goal-line football, championship boot hockey, or whatever his latest invention was. James always had an amazing imagination, the ability to create a situation, paint it for us like a picture, and make it all seem bigger than life. In this way, he is wonderfully contagious.

Today, James is married and a father of three. He runs his own law firm, is a fantastic cook, a lover of history, and fiercely competitive. He is a problem solver, a hard worker, and always a force to be reckoned with. He is my older brother.

Now you have met my family. We were an average family, perhaps happier than some but by no means perfect. But now, my memories travel through the lens of death and trauma. It changes my perception, makes me treasure things that I might not have otherwise—my father's hilariously stubborn tuft of hair or the playful bounce in my sister's step when she was laughing. These things are made more meaningful by the death that became their lives.

Death and trauma also bring questions. For starters, which family were we? An average one from a small city situated along Lake Superior's north shore, a family who happened into some bad luck; or were we never average and always headed down that embankment? Which?

A similar question shadows my own path. Has trauma brought me two lives: one as a walking person and another as a paralyzed one? Or has my life been a preparation for itself, for who I am now? Death and trauma reach through one's life with stunning swiftness.

It may seem that the car accident has led me to question fate, to wonder about destiny. Of course it has, but my interest is one of identity, both as a family and as an individual. What is identity in the face of a radical disruption? Who was I? Who am I? Who will I be? Truthful answers to these questions often take years and years to realize. This is true regardless of whether there is fate or whether there is a plan. To answer such questions, we need healing stories.

Healing trauma requires opening one's life to interpretation, creating a personal mythology to guide perception, and forging a set of healing stories that create or maintain a sense of identity.

Perceiving foreknowledge of one's fate is one way to do this. It is like saying, "See, I was here before you. I knew you were coming." Such a healing story gives a measure of control where there seems to be none. Somehow, if you can see a punch coming, it's better than being blindsided. We all experience mild versions of it, even in everyday life: "I was just thinking about you and you called," or "I had a feeling it was going to be a bad day." This longing for a connection deeper than random defines the human condition.

I am ten—three years before the accident. I am sleeping soundly in bed when my brother rousts me awake. Recently, we have begun to share a room—my mother believes it is the best way to ensure a lifetime of closeness. She is right. So his trip to my bed is a short one, but his voice is breathless. Across the room, his bed-side lamp shines—I can just make out his face. He is sitting on the floor with his knees pulled into his chest. He is rocking slightly, he has been crying.

"Matt, I couldn't find you. There was grass everywhere, tall grass, but you were nowhere."

"Huh?"

"No one else was around, just you and me, but I couldn't find you."

"James, what's wrong? You're scaring me."

"Something terrible happened. I can still feel it in my chest."

"It's just a bad dream. I'm right here."

"I know, but I couldn't find you."

This dream still haunts James and me to this day.

A year or so later, my brother's friend from junior high, some-one he hasn't seen for a couple years, calls and asks to come over. John has already started on a path that will lead him to become a Jesuit monk. As a consequence, he takes anything that feels prescient quite seriously—not an easy pressure on a young friend-ship. Visibly shaken, he tells my brother of a dream he had: Our family was in some kind of accident, someone died, and it felt so real. My brother, long out of the grip of his own dream, patiently listens but then sends John away, musing that his friend has gotten quite weird.

Eerie in retrospect, like seeing someone for the last time before something awful happens, these dreams left no lasting imprint—at least not until the accident happened.

There were also waking visions. My mother claims one as early as age twelve. There is a man whom she sees clearly, then an accident, and then a death, all coming in powerful flashes. Based on these visions, my mother comes to believe that she will die prematurely. Years later, she is twenty and driving with the man who will be my father. She identifies him with the earlier vision and wonders if she is to die soon. My mother has another vision, about a year before the accident. She is painting. She suddenly "sees" that she will have another lover—a strange thought for an incredibly devoted wife. She stops painting, sits down, and is seized with dread.

On Halloween night, just twenty-seven days before the accident, I make an outrageously ironic comment. I am courting Sheila, my first junior high school crush. The evening is full of rowdiness and fun, but also talking. I find out that she has an older brother who lives with a spinal cord injury. He is paralyzed from the chest down. As she tells me, I feel a powerful rush of sympathy, both because I feel like I stumbled into a family secret and for the life her brother is forced to live. I am so struck by what I imagine to be his experience that I say, "I'd rather be dead than in a wheelchair."

My sister approaches both my mom and some of her friends

and speaks of dying—this in the months just preceding her death. My Aunt Kathy, after adopting two children and trying to get pregnant for her entire adult life, quits smoking and accidentally conceives at the age of forty-one. Her child is born in April 1978, seven months before our crash. She unexpectedly names her little girl after my sister, Laura Kathleen. The second Laura Kathleen also dies young—at the age of twenty-three.

During my sister's sophomore year of college, she develops her own calligraphy. She copies, in black ink on gold paper, a stanza from a poem I do not know:

> Remember me,
>
> as I do you,
>
> with all tenderness
>
> which it is possible for one.

She makes three copies and gives them to my mother. One of these now hangs framed on my office wall. I look at her beautiful handwriting and wonder if this is what she intended.

I am not claiming anything about foreknowledge or about destiny. I am trying to prove nothing. These are simply instances thrown up by experience, from memory, that now take on heightened meaning. All can be explained in one way or another. Had we not tumbled down that embankment, these experiences would mean nothing and simply fall into the ever-receding pit of memory. But instead, they were brought forward by events and constructed into a mythology of healing stories that help my family feel a sense of control. This mythology was constructed sometimes for our comfort, sometimes to raise the hair on the back of our necks, but always to feel a connection to the life that was ours.

My life seems to have changed its course at least a few times— surviving the car accident at age thirteen, beginning to study Iyengar yoga twelve years later, and the birth of my twin sons nearly nine years after that. But I am no longer sure that this makes sense; I no longer feel changes of direction. Instead, as I grow older, I see a unity to the patterns of my life. I see that it has been feeding itself, like a river gaining current.

According to my mom, when I was two months old and she was patting my back to burp me, I began patting on her back in return. Rather than feeling the attention solely on me, I redirected it outward. When I awoke from a coma years later, rather than dwelling on my own devastation, I shifted my focus toward the needs of my remaining family—an intuitive move that probably saved my life.

As a kid, I was amazingly accident prone. Enduring a plethora of mishaps—requiring stitches four times and breaking two bones before reaching age ten—taught me something important about healing. How one handles pain and injury demonstrates character. Silly as it seems, my first inkling of this came when I was in the first grade. I was wearing my favorite pants—red corduroys with jamming metal studs along the side—and running full speed down the school playground's slide. I slipped on someone's spit and landed on my left knee. The result was a call to my mom, a trip to the emergency room, and three stitches. Rather than stay home and milk my mother for special attention, I chose to return to school, to show the other kids and especially my teacher that I was tough, that I could handle a little pain and return to life as usual. In retrospect, it feels like a blueprint for the future.

I had a particularly disastrous summer between third and fourth grades. I broke my foot falling off a six-foot-tall rock, I cracked the growth plate on my right knee jumping on a huge inner tube in our neighbor's driveway, and I deeply sliced my finger with a jackknife while on a family canoeing trip. I was proud of my list of injuries—they were like notches on my belt. My father didn't share my swelling pride and sat me down for a talk.

"I'm concerned, Matt," I remember my dad's face as hard but expressionless. "You're still a young kid and look what you've already done to your body. This summer you've been a walking disaster."

My gaze cast downward, I said, "I don't understand."

"Matt, you run around with your head in the clouds. Look at the consequences. You need to pay more attention; you need to look before you leap." A sly smile broke across my face. "It's not a laughing matter," he firmly commanded. "What if the accidents get bigger as you get bigger—more serious? What then?"

"What are you saying?"

"I want you to be more careful, to grow old and have a full life. You've got to use your head, or you might not make it."

Fear pulsed through me. My father spoke of something I

couldn't quite grasp, but I had an inkling. I didn't feel scared exactly, but I suddenly knew something had to change. "Dad, how can I control accidents? I don't understand . . ."

"Hopefully by being more aware," was his even response.

The world suddenly became bigger—I wasn't invincible. My own death was making its first conscious appearance in my world. It changed me; it vaguely changed the way I experienced my life. Something quiet had been added, something subtle, like another light in an already lit room. Remembering, I am struck by that conversation. It contained three defining features of my upcoming life—pain and injury, my response to it, and the possibility of death.

As I left my father's bedroom that day, my seeking path became a little more tangible. Did I have a vision of what lay ahead, of my upcoming experiences? Not really. But the feeling, the struggle to understand, the alertness that I took away from that encounter strike me now as a form of preparation, as a form of grace.

If life allowed it, I would go back and hold that boy, whisper to him, let him feel warmth before life breaks him apart. I love him in that moment, when he somehow senses an unpredictable future. I love his willingness to move forward, to engage, to use a strength that is born of innocence. Feeling without knowing, that is our fate.

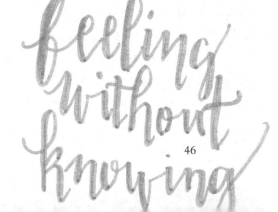

46

5

Pain and Silence

For well over three weeks, I have been surviving a waiting period in the intensive care unit. Waiting for when: when my condition stabilizes, when I can withstand more-aggressive treatment. Contrary to prime-time television dramas, hospitals are boring. They are not like the fast-paced, code-blue, blood-spurting images we watch while eating popcorn. Instead, surviving devastating trauma features an abundance of mind-numbing time. It requires incredible endurance, a timeless focus when nothing else is possible.

In particular, I am waiting for surgery. My back must be stabilized. The three vertebrae between my shoulder blades, T4–6, are severely displaced to the back and left. The procedure will be extensive, requiring six to eight hours and the stamina of two orthopedic surgeons. They will attempt to straighten my skewed spinal column, harvest bone from my hip, and then fuse the damaged vertebrae together. Finally, they will insert into my body two interlocking Harrington rods, with their accompanying nuts and hooks, along each side of my spine. These rods will span about seven vertebrae, from the base of my neck to my middle back.

They will stabilize my spine while the bone fusion solidifies, a process that takes about two years. As these large chunks of metal are submerged into my back, I feel like a tar pit, absorbing tubes, screws, IVs, needles, and now rods into the darkness of my body.

The surgery will be a good thing. The Foster frame has been only a resting place until I can survive the violence of this procedure. Being fit enough means I have made progress. More important, having surgery is the first step toward leaving this frame and entering a plaster body cast. I am promised that the cast will markedly curb my excruciating pain, a pain that is seemingly untouched by drugs.

I cannot say that this pain is consuming. That implies I have boundary enough to recognize my own consumption. I don't. This pain obliterates my cohesion, like pools of water separating on an uneven floor. It is not the acute pain of, say, breaking a wrist. Hurt as that does, the wrist is only a peripheral body part, not the core. It is possible to isolate your wrist, surround the pain, know its beginning, and foresee its end. The pain I have at this point grants no such luxury. It undercuts any unified sense of self, spreading me thinner and thinner—a silent hollowing toward death.

I remember nothing of the day of surgery, not the lead-up, not anything. Like the day of the car accident, there is a blotch in my continuity. Perhaps intense trauma reaches back into memory and erases what needs forgetting. Maybe it's like the precise moment one falls asleep—remembering its passage might reveal a necessary secret.

In any case, the surgery went well. The fusion took, the hardware was installed. A neurosurgeon was called in to take a look, but, as predicted, the damage was too extensive—nothing could be done to reverse my paraplegia. His confirming verdict: paralysis for all the days that I shall live. It is too early for disappointment, as I am barely holding it together. I am not able to think about anything yet, let alone the future. All I can do is tell myself, *This is things getting better.*

After a week or so, it is time for a body cast. How bad could it be? *It's just a cast,* I say to myself. I am hopeful, as though I am coming down the homestretch.

I am taken to an operating room. It is cold. Yellow tile is everywhere except overhead. Above is dominated by penetrating surgical lights. As I lie on my back, I see spots that shift as I move my eyes and are highlighted when they cross the shadowed faces of those around me. As this is not a sterile procedure and there are no surgical masks, I can see mouths move, even connect them to the voices bouncing off the tile. My gurney is lined up parallel to a bigger structure. It is a frame, like that of a canopy bed. But there is no mattress, just a platform of three metal bars running lengthwise. People close in around me. "One, two, three," someone says, and I am hoisted up onto this rack, a naked, shivering five-foot-six-inch body and a mind unprepared for what is coming. Since the surgery, my back is a screaming bundle of cut nerves and muscles, like kindling and gasoline waiting to ignite. The pressure of lying on three narrow metal bars is the match. A searing burn courses through me, my recently sewn flesh rages alarm. I become lost in the fire that is my back.

As the pain is literally unbearable, my mind escapes and becomes intensely aware of the smell of the room. It attempts to attach elsewhere, allowing only an edge of what's happening. It's not unlike admiring the beautiful sky of a sunset but not peering directly at the sun itself. The needed result: a nearly mindless body absorbs the unconscionable pain.

Time goes off-screen. When I come around, I am back in intensive care. I feel like I have been assaulted, subjected to a curious blend of betrayals. At least the drawn curtains are familiar. I am back where I started.

Just as things couldn't get worse, they get better. The pain has decreased. The plaster encases my whole torso, front and back, from my pubic bone, over my shoulders, and surrounding the base of my neck. The cast gives me boundaries, borders around the pain. The result is a calming compression, a feeling of safety that allows me to let go.

In retrospect, I realize how profoundly this feeling of boundary imprinted me. It is an insight that I will carry through my lifetime. Years later, a calming compression is what I experience when I practice yoga. (I now recognize it as the feeling of embodiment.) The spinal integrity of that thirteen-year-old boy was spewing all over the place, like a downed electrical line. The plaster cast directed this spillage back through his body, restoring his sense of place.

The body cast allows me to move off the Foster frame and into a bed. This is my Christmas present from Dr. McMeken, who insists that I be released from the intensive care unit. "Too long here makes anyone crazy, especially your family," he says. Dr. McMeken is a handsome Aussie, middle-aged, with blond hair, flaming blue eyes, and a mustache. I love hearing him talk. There is something so crisp and pure about an Australian accent. It inherently springs joy.

Moving me out of intensive care is a medically questionable decision, but Dr. McMeken works a compromise among all of my attending physicians. The plastic surgery ward has only four of its twenty-two beds occupied. Apparently, cosmetic surgery doesn't mix well with the holidays. Here I will get extra attention simply because they are overstaffed and the nurses need something to do. I lose the geese migration but gain an amazingly friendly nursing staff.

Dr. McMeken does something else for me, though. He gives me wonderful stories about Australia. He tells me about the color of the water, the night stars, the Great Barrier Reef, and the prevalence of great white sharks. But the snakes—we speak long and hard about the snakes. He grew up in the rural areas, where snakes, especially poisonous ones, are quite common. He claims that one should never walk off into the countryside in shorts but wear only long, thick pants. One should also carry a walking stick, not for support but for protection. I suspect that he is pulling my leg. Still, I make him describe all the different snake varieties, their coloring, their mannerisms. I even learn that his mother was the local expert at "flipping" snakes, whatever that means. His stories take me to a mysterious land with sharks and snakes but also with walking sticks, shimmering blue water, and exotic beauty. Do I know that the life ahead of me will be much the same, that going forward I will journey into a strange territory? Not exactly; I am only thirteen. But Dr. McMeken performs an essential healing task. He relights my imagination.

It's funny what can bring reprieve. A body cast makes obvious sense. The core of my body—the spine—is held firmly in alignment. My body's energy regains downward guidance to my feet. From the outside to in, from plaster to bone, I am held steady. Just as important, though, are these stories of Australia. Through my imagination, my perception begins to move. No longer just statically absorbing trauma after trauma, it shakes off and begins to light. I feel more hopeful because I start to "see" in color again. Now, I look forward to seeing people, not just being with them. I start to notice their moods, their footsteps, their mannerisms. I make jokes; I tease—all signs that the pain is becoming manageable. I need these connections because I am heading down another tunnel.

The upcoming trauma proves to be a defining one. But not because of its severity, or its overtly dramatic effect. Rather, how I responded was critical, how I prepared. It was my first conscious attempt to remove my mind from my body.

One day during their 6 a.m. rounds, the orthopedic residents tell me that my body cast isn't fitting right and that I need a new one. My mother arrives a couple of hours later. She enters softly, pulls the chair a little closer to my bed, and sits down lightly. Immediately, she sees that I am distraught. "What's wrong?"

"I need another body cast . . . Mom, I can't do it." Tears fall softly over her cheeks. How does a mother watch her little boy suffer again and again? She is desperate. A pivotal conversation ensues, the first of a series.

"Matt, tomorrow, try leaving your body for a while." She leans back and grabs the arms of her chair. Her posture reaches for authority as her gaze moves sideways into emptiness.

"What?"

"You're smart enough . . . just step outside the pain." Silence.

"So it's okay, then . . . just to let it happen?" I am vaguely afraid but also relieved.

"Yes."

"I know what you're talking about," my voice barely audible.

"Good." As an empty, dulled look claims my mom's face, I am forced to look away. She has moved past tears, toward silence, for the survival of her child.

I recognize the importance of this conversation primarily in retrospect. At the time, it seemed ordinary and practical, not strange and metaphysical. After all, the experience of moving out of my body was already occurring. Her words felt like a whisper in my ear, a granting of permission, a way to trust and let go.

Years later, I find out that her desperate advice came in part from a passage in Aldous Huxley's novel *Island*. A main character, enduring a painful death from cancer, leaves her body and watches from the corner. My mom has always explored ideas through books, and this time, she hit the mark straight on.

A very odd encounter also likely played a part. At about this time, Bob Hardman, the new minister from our church, paid my mother a visit. She had recently rejoined his church after a five-year hiatus. We had attended services only intermittently, so we knew him sketchily at best. He made the drive from Duluth and met privately with my mom. I never saw him.

"Paula, I have something a little awkward to tell you. I don't really believe that God talks to us through dreams, and yet I feel compelled." He fidgets but then continues, "I had a vivid dream the other day . . . I was told that Matt would pursue an alternative path, some alternative form of healing. You need to trust this, it's okay."

"Can you be more specific?" my mom asks.

"I can't. I am at a loss. I just know that I am to tell you." A strained pause. "This seems strange, I know, but I felt it was my duty to . . ."

"I am touched by your concern. Thanks for coming."

My mom does not tell me about this conversation for years, although it guides some of her actions. A few years later, she lets a friend pay for a psychic/astrologist to do an extensive chart on me. Years after that, when a friend recommends a body worker, she immediately puts us in contact. Finally, when I come home from graduate school and proclaim my lifelong commitment to the practice of yoga, she smiles and tells me about the strange visit with Bob Hardman.

And maybe, just maybe, this odd encounter led my mom to set the whole thing in motion, to offer her own interpretation of an alternative path. In the heat of the moment, she had reached back and pulled an image from her own idea of metaphysics and offered it to her desperately hurting child.

This conversation began my first conscious attempts to dislocate my mind from my body. It is not like I suddenly became an expert. But I did vaguely grasp that a resource existed within me, a silent place into which I could retreat and find protection. What I didn't realize was the long-term cost of going there and becoming comfortable.

The day quickly arrives for my second body cast. It's one thing to get mugged; it's even worse to know that you are going to get mugged. I am a mess—terrified, panicked, and silent.

It turns out that this next encounter with plaster is somewhat anticlimactic. I am prepared to go to war, to leave my body, to kick, to scream, to push back. The procedure is still painful, but nothing like before. Maybe my back has healed some. Perhaps I am gaining ground. In part, there is a practical explanation. My old cast is not sawed off me all at once; instead, it is done in sections. This means that the doctors replaster in segments, and my naked body does not press against that metal rack all at once. My back smolders but never completely catches fire.

I am getting better at this. I know that the trauma will not annihilate me, that my mind can find a silent place, and my body will absorb the pain. Within this silence, I am gaining confidence.

～

For Christmas, I receive a Bigfoot stuffed animal from a family friend. To this day, I've never seen one bigger. It sits five feet tall, its three-toed feet at least two feet high, its nose almost a foot long. Long, reddish brown hair and a goofy grin make for a hilarious appearance. The 1,200-bed hospital is relatively empty; my ward is down to three patients, and holiday spirits are running high. The nursing staff is so bored that the games begin. They admit Bigfoot as a patient, give him a private room next to mine, and create his own medical chart. They call staff members to draw blood, give IVs, and even catheterize him. They add him to the doctors' scheduled rounds and even get some to write orders and comments in his chart. There are many howls and giggles. Bigfoot is a hit. For me, it is the best part of this Christmas.

I am beginning to feel flashes of being a thirteen-year-old boy. I have a color television, complete with a remote control, neither of which we have at home. Better yet, no one tells me I can't watch late-night TV. Who would dare? Sleep does not come easy when one is in bed every hour of every day. So I stay up late, very late. This becomes a problem. Often, I do not wake up for the doctors' early-morning rounds. For a while I fool them, as I

have developed the habit of sleeping with my eyes open. This is
not great for the eyes, but it makes for more morning sleep. Unfortunately, the doctors catch on, and I am denied the television
flipper after 11 p.m. For a thirteen-year-old, this feels like being
held hostage.

Why don't they understand how hard the nights are? Alone, in
the dark, and unable to sleep is when my new reality envelops me.
I do anything I can to avoid it. My brother gives me a red-lighted,
hand-controlled electronic football game, and I play it well into the
night. Sometimes a night nurse named Ray plays it with me. Those
nights are less painful. Soon, I will be denied access to this, too.
Apparently they think I need more sleep—as if it were that easy.

My friend Roger has given me a tape recorder. The idea is that
we can send tapes back and forth. He sends me a tape of him talking while he puts on his equipment for a hockey game. His life is
so different from mine. I never get focused enough to send one
back. But the tape recorder serves a different purpose for me. My
brother tapes a cassette with Jackson Browne's *Running on Empty*
and Jerry Rafferty's *City to City* on it. I feel grown up, sharing
music with my brother. I identify with the title track of the first
album in the dramatic way that only a thirteen-year-old can. It is
exactly how I feel. I am running on empty, and I am old enough
to know. The second album was my sister's favorite when she
died. She had played "Baker Street," the album's best track, many
times, helping me feel how the lone, dreamy saxophone carries
the song. I listen to this tape over and over as I silently and unconsciously grieve in the institutional darkness.

There is a man who often comes and breaks the monotony of

my nights. He is on the "cath" team, a group of people who go from room to room "cathing" the needy. This means that he inserts a sterile catheter into my penis and pushes it through my urethra into my bladder. The force of gravity then drains the urine into a measuring container. When he comes, I am usually quite drowsy. The encounter is often dreamlike.

The light from the hallway shines brightly around his imposing body. The cathing process takes about ten minutes, leaving plenty of time to fill. One night I notice his forearms. At first I think it is just the relative darkness, but then I realize that he has incredibly hairy arms. I start to take more notice. Where he stops shaving on the underside of his chin, about from his Adam's apple down, he is solid hair—no skin visible at all. This is an incredibly hairy man! Or is he? As the nights wear on, I begin to imagine, or dream, or whatever the state is, that I am being cathed by an ape. At first this image is funny, but after a while it begins to spook me. Now when he comes, I insist that he turn on the room light. I need to see him. The sighting is confirmed: This *is* the hairiest man I have ever seen.

So begins our speaking relationship. I make him show me his ankles and calves—solid hair. Turns out that this ape-man is also a great storyteller. I particularly like his cathing war stories. He once cathed a truck driver who had 4,500 cc of urine in his bladder—that's four and a half quarts. Can you imagine all the times that man denied himself the relief of peeing?

Imagine this, imagine that. I collect stories, from Dr. McMeken, from the ape-man, from anyone who is willing to share. Anything to hold my wonder . . . the nights wear on.

6

Mind, Not Body

It is mid-January. Night and day bring only more waiting. This time I am waiting for my bones to heal. Both my neck and my back need to take hold, to throw down enough new calcium to support themselves. Until this happens, movement is risky, sitting up isn't possible, neither is rehabilitation. So we wait—the three of us—my mind, my body, and the silence as waves of trauma continue to break along my shores.

When I turn my focus inward toward my paralyzed body, I feel no inside, no connection, nothing. There is no evidence that I am "in" there at all. It's so different from when I look at my hand. In my hand, there is a sense of immediate presence. The connection between my intent and my hand manifests as movement. So intimate is the connection that it seems built into the very fabric of having a body. Not so when my mind reaches downward toward my legs. Rather than an immediate connection, my paralyzed body presents a brick wall. So abrupt, so foreign, the perceived absence of sensation is enough to make me nauseous.

This is yet another level of greeting the silence. I am now

living in a body that presents silence rather than tangible sensation. When the nurses turn me from side to side, I do not feel my ankle bones knock together. I do not feel the warmth of my inner thighs touching or the comforting weight of the sheet draped over me. Within much of my body, what I have known as living has been replaced by a resounding silence.

This silence that I perceive within my body came upon me abruptly through a spinal cord injury. For most people, however, the process is slower. It develops through aging. Over time, the body becomes slower to respond, more likely to sit at rest, more content to observe rather than act. But in each case, the fundamental healing question remains the same: What aspect of consciousness will traverse the increasing gap between mind and body? The answer will depend upon our healing stories.

Through the medical model, I will encounter one kind of healing story. My rehabilitation will guide me to willfully overcome this new silence. In my case, it will not suffice.

In the short term, however, I take a very practical approach to this silence. I use the dislocation between my mind and body as a means of protection. I hear silence where there is pain. I embrace my neurologically induced rupture.

I target the IVs. I am so sick of them: the incessant pricks and pokes of needles, the hardened and painful skin around a long-lasting IV site, the constant hair-pulling from the tape holding them in place, the sting of new drugs dripping into my bloodstream. Thus far, the IVs have always been inserted into my hands and arms, but now these veins are refusing to cooperate. They have hardened, become wiry, and literally sunk deeper into my body. I am both tickled and saddened by their ingenuity—my body is fending for itself. But then it strikes me. How about the veins in my feet? Why not stick me down there? The medical vampires oblige; they too are frustrated and willing to try anything. I gain a much-needed reprieve. Blood draws and IVs don't happen to me down there. They affect that other body, the silent one. I feel clever, like I am pulling a fast one.

Unfortunately, the veins in my feet prove to be no dumber than the ones in my arms. Over time, they too begin to hide successfully. I am presented with two options: Use my arms again or have my head shaved and begin using my scalp. I feel punished as the digging resumes in my arms. I am disappointed by my worthless feet.

〜

The orthopedic doctors just won't stop. Mainly, I deal with two fourth-year residents. Dr. Quinlan is an officer in the Army Reserve. She has short black hair, plainly cut. Small, wire-rimmed glasses surround hard brown eyes. Her upper lip barely moves when she speaks, as if she is clenching her jaw. This mirrors an absence of gestures—her arms are seemingly fastened to her sides. She is not attractive, nor is she unattractive, and seems to desire neither. She is a tough woman who embodies military discipline.

Dr. Basset is a balding weight lifter. Slightly pigeon-toed, a big smile, and even bigger arms, he obviously loves what he does. He reminds me of a boy playing grown-up. One day he tells me he can bench-press 390 pounds—I imagine the Incredible Hulk. Dr. Basset wants to fix the bones in my wrist. Apparently, the break in my left wrist was severe. Both he and Dr. Quinlan believe that it was set improperly and must be rebroken. I am assured that I won't feel a thing. They will pinch a nerve in my armpit and my arm will temporarily become part of my paralyzed body.

The first time the pinching doesn't work. The bone breaking will have to be rescheduled. I am not bothered; I will not feel anything anyway. The next time it works, and I lose the "inside" connection to my arm. They saw off my cast and also remove the splint from my right wrist. They want to take x-rays of both. Finally, I get to the operating room. I realize that I must have been given Valium because this feels strange but not frightening.

Dr. Quinlan approaches and tells me that my left wrist must be put in traction, to lengthen it before rebreaking it. She brings in a stand with what looks like Chinese handcuffs suspended from a horizontal metal bar. Each of my fingers is inserted into a finger cuff. My arm hangs downward from the fingertips, its weight providing the necessary traction for my wrist. She leaves. I am left alone, lying flat on my back, my unfelt arm hanging from a wire contraption that looks like a form of torture. The Valium must be helping. The picture strikes me as absurd. Inwardly laughing, I drift off into a light sleep.

I awaken to multiple bodies around me. I do not recognize the doctor who has my wrist. He is cranking it in awkward directions, yanking, twisting, doing anything to gain the desired break. He is unsuccessful. He tells me that once the body recalcifies a fracture, the bone becomes stronger than before, making resetting it more difficult. Dr. Basset's physique is called in. But his ability to bench-press nearly 400 pounds is no match for the scrappy, healing bones of my thirteen-year-old body. At one point, he puts his leg over my wrist in an attempt to gain better leverage. He yanks hard upward. I see the muscles straining in his arms; I even detect sweat. Still nothing. My wrist is holding firm. By this point, I am laughing. The movie in front of me could not be better scripted.

I hear whispering off to my right, little snippets: "His other wrist isn't healing straight. It needs resetting." Another voice says, "But if we reschedule, it will take time. The longer we wait, the worse it gets." I am still watching Dr. Basset's futile struggle with my left wrist. Somebody quietly grabs my right arm. Out of the corner of my eye, I see a sudden twist. A horrible cracking, more like a shattering, echoes through the room. On an exhale, "You fucking broke my wrist!" The pain blindsides me. "Who the fuck are you people! I can't believe you broke my other wrist . . ." My voice quickly trails off into sobs and wails of unsuspected betrayal. Vaguely, I hear someone tell me that the cast will ease the pain. In furied silence, I watch as they form casts on both my wrists: one that refused to break and one that was tricked. The pain eases, but it's too late. I trust no one.

Back in my room, hatred is not quite what I feel. I am beyond not trusting the doctors, beyond thinking I possess clever resources. I feel little and helpless and naked. I have to be ready for anything, from any direction. If they can break my wrist without anesthesia, then anything is possible. I withdraw and move inward. Although silence remains a tool, a perceptual buffer, it now becomes a place to stay, a place to wait. It envelops me. My body becomes seamless, the backs of my eyes ache with emptiness but also begin to flicker with a different kind of strength. Part of my living dies so I can continue forward. I move farther away from my body.

Take a breath, hold it, feel how the silence invades from all sides, how things become just a little more still. That's what I am doing. I am riding motionless waves, holding myself thinner and thinner, making less of me for them to break, growing tougher through the silence.

⌒

Every day, all day, I lie in bed. So stale, not just the smell but the dullness, the lack of change, the lack of freshness. My only measure of control is throwing off the sheet that covers me. Just increasing the amount of air touching my skin can bring temporary relief, or so I wish. I begin to throw off the sheet more and more often and think nothing of it. Any control of my environment feels like a victory. I continue this practice for a period of time, perhaps weeks.

On this weekend, both my brother and Bob are visiting. They have been to a movie—*Invasion of the Body Snatchers,* the recent remake with Donald Sutherland. They enter my room bubbling; obviously the distraction has been good for them. Knowing that life continues outside of my room, that there are still theaters and popcorn and Junior Mints, seems a necessary thing, proof that the world still holds fun. Hearing about it feels like food.

"How was it?" I ask. They pause, fidget from foot to foot.

"Good," Bob finally replies.

"Come on, give me more than that."

"Why don't you pull the sheet up?" my brother asks.

"Why?" He and Bob look at each other and burst out laughing. "What's so funny?" I ask.

"Just that it's hard to keep a straight face when . . ." Bob's voice stumbles, "when you're lying there naked like that." His words pour out awkwardly.

"Matt, you're sharking us right now."

"Baring it all, as they might say," Bob chirps in.

"I am not! My cast is covering me."

"No, it's not," my brother says, his gaze cast downward.

"Yeah, it is." Confidently, I reach for my groin. "Oh my god." Sting rushes across my face like getting hit with a basketball. As I touch around my penis for the first time in months, I feel something strange. "James, is that pubic hair?" Tears stream from everywhere. I feel sick. "Why didn't you tell me?"

"I thought you knew." My brother steps closer, kneels next to the bed. "It's okay."

During my short three months in the seventh grade, the locker room called forth one of life's painful unfoldings. Showering after gym hadn't been too difficult, because other kids also lacked any sign of puberty—there was safety in numbers. But showering after basketball practice was different. I was the only seventh grader on the ninth-grade varsity team, a babe in the hormonal woods. Acutely aware of this, I longed for the changes ahead, for the time when I would begin the path toward physical manhood, for the time when I would join the others.

Instead, my rite of passage is a public viewing—for everybody and without my knowledge. How could I not know it was happening, not sense something, anything? Rather than pride and feelings of becoming, there is only embarrassment—my body's changing innocence is exposed to everyone, from the candy striper offering magazines to the woman who cleans my room. But I can go nowhere, escape to nowhere. My only option is to silently absorb. I am without power, without pride, and now without dignity.

I feel de-spirited. It feels pointless to have a body. This is the problem with the silence gaining such a strong foothold: It can just as easily fuel a sense of loss, purposelessness, or even depression. Although silence lies at the center of wonder and appreciation, even strength, it also can breed powerlessness, indifference, and apathy. Robbed of my passage into puberty, I become less and less interested in having a body at all.

ᔕ

66

I am ripe for healing stories that guide me away from my body. It is where I want to go. A man in the room next to mine is lonely and a high-level quadriplegic. One day my mom goes over for a visit.

Upon her return, she looks rattled. It turns out that he is in his mid-twenties and lives in a nursing home. Incapable of movement below his neck, he describes a life of complete and utter dependency. He has a tough life, and his sadness unintentionally paints a dismal picture of living with a spinal cord injury. He leaves my mother with a powerful parting image: "I feel like a floating head."

My mom and I are in a vulnerable position. We have no idea what living with paralysis will actually be like. Will I also feel like a floating head? We do at least know that my situation is different from his. I am a paraplegic, not a quadriplegic. I will be able to use my arms, to feed myself, even drive a car someday. Yet, despite these differences, his image is haunting.

My mom returns to visit me the next day. She impresses upon me another pivotal healing story after having struggled through a sleepless night.

"Matt, there are a lot of differences between you and the man next door."

"I know. We talked about them yesterday."

"More than that. He is a very nice man, but he's not very educated. Smart enough, but nothing shining." She pauses to see if I follow. My look is blank. "What I'm trying to say is that when he lost his body, he lost his best resource. That's not true about you."

She pauses again and stares straight ahead. Her voice trembles, "I know you loved playing sports more than anything . . . you were so good at them. But Matt, you're also a very bright boy. School has always come so easily. Do you know how lucky you are?"

"I guess so." I feel anxious, like I'm being told that I will like brussels sprouts.

"Your mind is what matters now. You need to know this. Certain things are no longer options . . . playing professional sports, being a carpenter, a manual laborer. You know—things that depend on your body. The truth is, you wouldn't have done these things anyway." She turns and makes eye contact. "Do you know what I mean?"

"I think so." What she's saying feels important; I need to "get" it. I reach without fully understanding and simply accept. "I need to do well in school, right?"

"Yes, and concentrate on developing your mind."

With this healing story, my mom offers a way to think about the rest of my life. I must move into my head and make my mind shine. Of course, this exactly matches what I want. My body feels foreign and full of pain. Things constantly go wrong with it, and it is even growing pubic hair without me. Being told that my future resides in my head, that it is my best resource, gives me permission to leave my body behind. I will move away from it and lead with my mind. That is what I will do.

Of course, none of this is exactly conscious. I do not suddenly decide, *Okay, I am my mind and not my body.* Instead, the drift is more subtle, slower. I pay more attention to my visitors, pay even more attention to the nurses. I let my body be turned from side to side; I do not participate. I stop listening to discomfort. I inwardly hold my breath and look outward, away from my body.

Take a moment to clench your jaw. Feel how this subtly separates the eyes, the gaze, the intent from the rest of the body. That is what I am doing. My body, especially my paralyzed body, continues to become an object. I judge it rather than connect to it. I leave it rather than feel it. This only deepens my sense of separation. It also gives me better access to anger and disgust. Both are effective ways "out" of body. Ask an anorexic.

⌒

I need anger. I need something, anything, because I am terrified. The screw above my right ear has become infected. The surrounding tissue burns and itches, but I shouldn't have told anyone. Now they're going to change it—remove the old screw, find another spot, and twist more metal into my skull. I am expecting a trip to an operating room, something to acknowledge what's coming. But there is no need, I am told. The doctor will do it right in my room, right in my bed. This is not a memory that I want where I sleep, but I am not in charge of venue. I am given a dose of Valium and made to wait. When the doctor arrives, my mom has to leave. She cannot witness what lies ahead for her youngest child. She will return afterward to pick up the pieces.

I notice that the doctor is carrying a regular toolbox. "Is that what I think it is?" I ask.

"Sure is," he replies with a smile. "See, it's no big deal. We even use a plain old screwdriver, courtesy of good old Mr. Stanley." He is trying to lighten the mood. It's not working. What am I to do? Where will I go? My jaw tightens; an angry focus takes hold. I'm leaving. I lose track of his words as I work to move somewhere else. He is at the side of my head. Warmth begins to touch my ear.

"See, that wasn't so bad. The infected screw is already out," he says with feigned cheerfulness. I focus my gaze on the lights overhead. I reach with inner-intent and pull and merge and pull and merge. Soon it starts: the bleeding, the tearing, the sound, the pressure, the cracking, and then there is nothing but the lights. I am the lights. I see nothing. I am pushed outward and wait for space enough to return.

I vaguely hear the words "All done." I can see in front of me again. The doctor is holding my arm; his voice attempts to soothe. I am ready for him to leave. My mom returns expecting pieces, but there are none. There is only an unclenching jaw and an angry silence. I am powering down and getting sleepy.

I awaken to my mom's steadfast presence. Her imploring,

heartbroken eyes ask, "Are you all right?" My first words, "I made it, Mom. I'm okay."

The old screw site is left open to heal. It doesn't. Later that evening, I feel around the wound. It stings. I feel remnants of dried blood, my hair feels caked, but there is also something else. Something is sticking out. I ask my mom for a hand mirror. I see what looks like a miniature canine erection—something red and angry—poking out of the side of my head. Neither my mom nor the nurses know what to make of it. The resident on call eventually comes. He is jovial and honest and says, "I've never seen anything like this. Most likely, this is the sac that surrounds your brain. It looks inflamed and is probably infected, causing it to seep out." He practices a commonsense remedy. He puts Vaseline over the site and wraps my head tightly with gauze. "Hopefully, this will push it back in." He tells me to have my regular doctors check it in the morning.

I am reminded of a Sven and Ollie joke my brother once told me. Sven falls asleep in the outhouse. Meanwhile, Ollie kills and guts a deer, then leaves the innards next to his unsuspecting brother. Sven finally returns to the house, visibly upset. He tells Ollie, "It was horrible; I woke up and found that I had plumb vomited out my innards. But with a little help from God and a stick, I was able to put them back in."

Not my intestines, but my brains leaking out the side of my head. Not God and a stick, but petroleum jelly and cloth. Once I get past the horror, a dark humor takes hold, a mixture of anger, submission, and absurdity. I can only silently observe the strange catastrophe that has become my body.

7

Gin and Tonics

There is another story, one I haven't been telling. Since the accident, my stomach, my intestines, my pancreas, almost everything in my digestive system has fallen completely silent, not a rumble, not a groan, not even a yawn. I cannot digest anything and have not eaten a morsel of food in nearly two months.

Each day the stethoscope moves under my cast, and each day the doctors say nothing. Although I am only marginally aware of the threat—back in 1979, people could not live indefinitely when being fed only through IVs—my mother and the attending doctor are very aware of it. Amazingly, Dr. Telander and my mom went to high school together. He is a pediatric internal medicine specialist. His belief is that my pancreas has been injured, which, in turn, has thrown everything else off-line. For sure, my pancreas had been recklessly pouring digestive juices in many places where it shouldn't. Recently that subsided, and they removed the tube running through my nose and down to my stomach. But still my body cannot take in food, not without causing irreparable harm.

I just assume that I will eat again; that's what living people do.

Unknown to me, though, as my mom walks from her motel to my bedside, she prays for rumblings in my stomach, for the beginnings of movement. For without them, I will die. One day I ask Dr. Telander what he is doing to help me eat again. He says there is nothing he can do. The body is its own best healer, and we must give my digestive system time.

I am obsessed with food. I miss the smell of my mom's baking bread, the taste of my birthday dinner roast beef, and the water burst in one of my grandma's homegrown tomatoes. Most of all, I miss the colors—eating colors, tasting colors, colors with nourishing dimension. This is to say nothing of what surrounds the act of eating. The shape of plates, the clanking of silverware, ice clinking from water pitcher to glass, the gathering of people, contact and love, all topped with food. People are at their best when they eat together. I miss it.

My longing is made worse by television. Bombarded by images of food every fifteen minutes, I start channel surfing for food commercials, especially for the perfect red of a diced tomato. The tomatoes in fast-food commercials are killer. Did I mention tomatoes? Did I mention the dirt in my grandma's immense garden, the sweat around the neck of her farm dress, the smell of noon dinner tucked within the dwarfing aroma of exposed earth? Did I mention what it was like to visit my grandparents' farm, the importance of lemonade on a hot summer day, the feeling of plucking a tomato off a ripening vine?

I am flooded by fantasies of food, by memories, the befores and afters, not even the actual meals. One second I am watching a perfectly made Big Mac, a price flashing yellow beneath the tempting treat. I don't need the cost; I need the burger. The next instant I am with my family. We are in the Boundary Waters Canoe Area, the Lower Forty-Eight's last bastion of wilderness, thankfully preserved in northern Minnesota. We are camping on an island; the sun is setting, the temperature dropping. Dessert is being made—dehydrated blueberry cobbler—just add boiling water and stir. I hear the methodical rubbing of tin spoon against tin bowl. I watch as liquid solidifies into goo. My mom opens the packet of crushed graham crackers, pours it on top, and pains me with the instruction that I must wait for it to cool. This will be the best dessert I have ever had. Suddenly, a car salesman is yelling at me, his cheap suit and bad hair shocking me back into my hospital bed. I still haven't eaten.

I become fixated on the restaurants surrounding the hospital. My visitors are always going out to dinner. It gets my mom away from the hospital and into a version of normal time. When they return—my mom, my brother, or whomever—I must know what they've eaten. Often I don't get past the first course. My mind has become stuck on the reddish orange, honeyed sweetness of Best Western salad dressing, especially when combined with the crisp, watery crunch of iceberg lettuce. I study faces, look for ever-so-slight smudges of grease, for toothpicks, for anything. I like it when a visitor has a beard. Sometimes, if I am lucky, there is a morsel left in a tuft of hair. I begin to guess what people have eaten by their expressions, by how they hold their bodies. Slow movements, touches of the belly, and unexpected exhales almost certainly mean a big piece of beef; self-righteous smiles usually imply some sort of salad; garlic belches become synonymous with pasta. My favorite restaurant is Michael's, a fancy steakhouse. I like how it smells on my people.

I have regrets. Some are easy to understand. I should have had another helping of stuffing. I should have been more thankful for my mom's meatloaf or for the sparse school lunches she made me—a cheese sandwich and a pear, there's nothing wrong with that. Oh, chocolate milk; I spend a lot of time thinking about stirring Nestle's Quick into a cold glass of Bridgeman's skim milk. More, I should have had more.

Other regrets are mysterious. I am caddying for my dad. The day is hot and I am starving. The ninth-hole concession stand sells hot dogs. I want two, but I am saving for a new putter. I buy an orange pop, one dog, and opt not to add any relish. No relish! What was I thinking? For some reason, I return to this memory over and over. Maybe it was the texture of the day, how the sun hit my face, or the way the strap of my father's golf bag cut into my shoulder . . . who knows what holds memory. As I lie here, all I know is that eating just one unrelished hot dog was a huge mistake.

My trauma-induced fast transforms my body from a healthy, athletic five foot six and 119 pounds to a taut, sunken shell of a boy weighing all of 80 pounds. Then one day—just like that—the rumblings in my stomach return. A medical student makes the discovery. He is bearded, with dark olive skin and thick glasses. His eyes light up; he pulls the stethoscope out of his ears and turns quickly to get the doctor. The rumbling is confirmed. My digestion has turned itself back on, from silence into function. My God, this means food. "*When can I eat?* I already know what I'm having!" "Not so fast," they say. "You need to start slow. It's clear liquids for you."

Bent straws, bent straws, and more bent straws. This is not eating. Clear liquids mean chicken broth, beef broth, and an assortment of Jell-O. I know that I should be happy, that I need to be patient. But this is not a hot dog with extra relish, ketchup, and mustard. That's what I'm having by the way—that long-lost hot dog from summers past. I will have to wait more than a week.

When it finally arrives, it is freezer-burned and without relish. It does not connect me to my previous life. As I set aside the promise of this hot dog on my hospital tray, I ache with the feeling that the path ahead of me will be unfamiliar, that I will be entering a very different world.

I have an experience that I cannot shake, a hallucination really. Every so often, I ask my mom for a hand mirror to survey how I look. I stare at the silver halo around my head, at the metal screws that puncture my temples. The surrounding skin falls inward like water circling a drain. The oddity of it all. Screws don't belong in someone's head, nor was my skull ever intended to provide backing for hardware. And yet, there it is.

My hair grows longer and longer. It's darker and very greasy, leaving marks on the pillow. My cheekbones stick out as the imposed famine has sucked my face inward. Dark rings sink beneath my eyes. I am painfully pale. My first acne shows on my forehead and new facial hair is threatening to connect my eyebrows. In the mirror, I see a boy who is beginning puberty—I do not recognize him. The decay that I am perceiving accelerates, moving past life and into a death mask. My bushy eyebrows are a straight line across my forehead, no shape to my face, just a pale skull and hair . . . my skin a colorless disappearing. I shudder with the feeling that I am seeing into my death. Just as quickly, the face I know returns and the apparition vanishes.

The time has come to move from the plastic surgery ward to the rehab floor. The descent is only from the third floor to the ground level, and I can even keep the same bed. But to me, it feels like I am going to another planet. I am leaving the security of my first home and moving to another. I feel like a baby bird falling from its nest. Everything about this new place feels different—the smell, the color of the lights, the shape of my room, everything. I lose my favorite nurses—Diane, Deloris, and Ray. I also lose Dr. McMeken, the strength behind his eyes, and the charming freshness of his smile. My new lead doctor is from Iceland. I can hardly understand him because of his accent; the words roll off his tongue at unusual pitches. He offers me no stories of an exotic land. Rightly or wrongly, the idea of Iceland brings me only images of desolate tundra. Unlike Australia, it does nothing to light my imagination. I feel both betrayed and strangely afraid.

I am introduced to my new lifelong companion: a wheelchair. The first one I sit in is burnt orange and has a back that is taller than my head. I need something to lean against because my neck can barely support weight. The chair is reclined to a forty-five-degree angle because if I sit up any more than that, I will faint. I am far too weak to push my own chair, but if I hold the IV stand, my mom can push me up and down the hallway. My endurance for sitting up is limited, so my stays in the chair are short, maybe fifteen minutes.

I was expecting more. I thought sitting up in a wheelchair would feel like a giant leap forward, that I would feel more like a person and less like a broken body. But the wheelchair does not bring reprieve. Instead, I feel unnatural and awkward, like a flustered guest. The experience is painfully unsettling.

I am told of a break room down the hall from my new room. It has a television that is equipped with video games. This catches my attention. I am excited at the prospect. My mom, however, is not much for video games. Rather than play with me, she sits and sketches in her notebook. Playing these games by myself is lonely and exposes them as pointless. Staring into a TV screen and pressing a button to shoot missiles at images of airplanes only heightens my feelings of emptiness and disconnection.

This is the silence rushing forward, the price of befriending it. While it has protected me, the silence has also put a distance between my actions and finding joy in things. I used to love playing video games. My neighbor had the first-generation home video game called Pong—we played it for hours at a time. But while playing these new games in the hospital, I feel nothing. I am shaken by the sense of not recognizing myself, like suddenly feeling lost in a familiar place. I want to say that the world has changed and it is to blame, but I know better. I have lost something, something invisible. I stop playing video games.

This is a moment familiar to most of us, a time when life suddenly becomes different, like the day when getting kissed by a parent is no longer comfortable or skipping no longer feels cool. In such examples, childhood innocence is discarded—for example, the act of skipping—so that something else can be embraced; that is, wanting to be a "bigger" kid.

When I stopped playing video games, something happened, something more akin to growing old. I had nothing with which to replace video games. Rather, I simply accepted the feeling of disconnection, of not feeling what I used to feel. I flatly accepted this loss of myself and stepped more deeply into the silent place between mind and body. The effect was deadening. This is an instance where the absence of a healing story is itself a healing story, although not a very good one. The silence was left to fester. The same thing occurs if we fail to stay present as we move into old age.

⌁

For the last few weeks, my brother has been talking to me, trying to convince me of something. "Matt, you've got to beat this thing," he whispers in quiet moments. "You have to believe you can beat the odds, that you will walk again." I try to believe him.

I cannot imagine what he feels when he is with me. We have spent so much time wrestling, playing, and imagining together. I have been working to follow in his footsteps for years, especially athletically. I have gotten a jump start on every sport possible. I have spent my childhood competing with older kids, honing my skills as he discovers them. I am a gifted athlete, and he has forged a clear path. Now he looks at me and struggles with acceptance— my body will never be the same.

One day I announce to Dr. Quinlan that I most definitely will walk again. The assertion is met with a frowning silence. Eventually, she admits that anything is possible, but that the odds are better that we will get hit by a meteor. She encourages me not to think about my condition in these terms.

This conversation concerns my doctors. They begin worrying that I might not be "accepting my situation," that I might be "harboring false hopes." In response, they keep reiterating the fact that my spinal cord has been severed, that I should plan on never walking again, and that I will experience no sensation below the level of my injury.

The last part confuses me, however. At first, when I tried to feel within my paralyzed body, I felt nothing. In fact, the acute absence of any sensation within my perception was alarming. But now, as I listen more carefully, as my condition improves enough for me to do so, I do feel something. It's not like normal sensation, like what I feel in my arms, for instance. But all the same, it is noticeable: tingles, surges, sometimes even mild burning. I tell the doctors. They grimace, worried that I will continue with what they perceive as denial. They prepare a powerful and pivotal healing story, one that aims to rid me of any false hope.

"Matt, what you are experiencing are phantom feelings," Dr. Quinlan explains. "You know, like ghosts or spooks. They're not real."

"Where do they come from then?" I ask.

"We don't know exactly. The best guess is that they are memory. Your mind remembers feeling your legs and continues to project their presence, even when they're not there." Her finger pushes her glasses securely back on her nose.

"Are you sure? They seem to be there even when I'm not thinking about them."

"Phantom feelings are widely reported by people who suffer an amputation. Lying in bed, they swear they still have two legs and are horrified to discover otherwise. The feelings can continue for quite a while. Some people even report them as downright painful. They are more of an annoyance than anything else. Luckily, as the mind forgets, these imagined sensations will fade."

"So I'm feeling what an amputee feels?"

"Yes."

Not the best healing story. Comparing my paralyzed legs to amputated ones only heightens my sense that they have become pointless. The silence within my perception grows deeper. Something in me riles with defensive pain. It's not easy to be told that what you are feeling isn't real. The healing story continues the next day.

"Dr. Quinlan, how do you know that what I'm feeling are phantom feelings?"

"Trust me, I know."

"How?"

"Experience. I just don't want you to think they mean anything . . . that they might be the beginning of walking again. Because they aren't. They aren't real." I feel pressed and getting angry.

"How do you know?" I snap.

"Okay, let's back up. Would you like to speak to a neurologist? Tell him about these feelings and then get examined?"

"Thank you, I would like that." Somehow, I feel vindicated.

Cometh the hammer. Not one but two neurologists enter my room. They look young, so they must be residents. I tell my story. They listen patiently and say, "Well, let's check it out." They have come prepared. A black case appears. Its contents include various needles, rubber mallets, and small hammers, some with rollers, some with spikes. "We use these things to test sensation. Don't worry, none of this will hurt." First, they test my arms. They poke my finger with a needle, run the roller hammer over my upper arm, show me the reflex in my elbow. Next they move to my feet and repeat the tests. "Are you feeling any of those sensations, any changes?" they ask. I am quiet. "How about this?" I say nothing. "I just stuck your toe hard enough to make it bleed and you didn't feel anything?" Again, silence. "Do you want us to show you again?" I am feeling sick and fighting back tears of humiliation. "See, whatever you are feeling is not connected to anything. The sensations are not real. They exist only in your head. We're sorry." These doctors are setting my reality picture. They seal the healing story with shame. Now I am an object of pity. They leave. Stupid boy, what were you thinking?

I do not feel bad for long. I simply believe them. The profound consequence of this healing story is practical: I stop listening to what is left of my mind-body relationship. No longer will I work to perceive anything from my paralyzed body. I accept that there is not and cannot be any remaining sensation, plain and simple. I actually feel silly to have thought otherwise. I move farther from my body and deeper into the silence.

The phantom-feelings healing story had an immediate impact. I was a good kid, trying to work through what I was told. It led to the following conversation.

"Mom, I've been thinking. My arms need to get really strong, right? If they have to do the work for both my arms and my legs, wouldn't it make sense if I didn't have legs? If they were amputated?" My mom sits in stunned silence. "My arms wouldn't have so much to carry. I'd be better off. I mean . . . since my legs can't help me anymore anyway, I could just lighten the load, couldn't I?"

"But Matt . . ." What do you say to a boy who is trying to jettison two of his limbs because it seems more functional? "You can't do that."

"Why? It makes sense."

"Because it's your body."

Such a notion doesn't even faze me. My mind has set upon a solution. This feels like moving forward. I ask my doctor.

"You don't want to do that," he replies.

"Why not?"

"Having your legs amputated is no little thing. It can never be undone. It's the only body you will ever have."

"So. I'm not going to need my legs," I say confidently. I have learned my part well. "Look, I'm trying to figure out my life. If my body weight is less, I will be more agile, better able to get around. It makes sense." The doctor sees my determination and tries a different tack.

"No, it doesn't. Having legs is critical for sitting balance, especially for you, since you lack any abdominal control."

"What do you mean?"

"Balance is going to be a challenge for you without the muscles in your stomach. Your legs will provide the necessary counterweight and make sitting easier. What if you reach for something while sitting in your wheelchair? What's going to keep you from falling onto the floor?"

"My legs?" I ask.

"Absolutely. See, you need them."

Not until this moment did I realize that my stomach muscles were also paralyzed. It never dawned on me. I have yet to sit up, roll over, or move around in bed. I haven't yet reached for anything from my wheelchair. Nothing. There has been no need to use my stomach muscles. I just assumed that they worked. I feel sick. My sense of disconnection from my body grows deeper, even alarming. How could I have not known something so basic? I'm paralyzed from the chest down. Of course that includes my abdominal muscles. What was I thinking? The good news is that I now grasp why I need to keep my legs attached to my body. It's a funny healing story: counterweight.

I have lost my childhood, and I know it. I tell people that I am thirteen going on forty-one—another healing story. I mean it. I have lost two-thirds of my body, the joy of video games, and much of my identity. What I have gained is the knowledge that I am older, that I must push forward and make it work. I want a rite of passage. I need acknowledgment.

My mind wanders to summers past. On warm nights, my mom and dad would sometimes sit on the patio drinking gin and tonics. I loved the smell, the color of the lime, and the sound of ice cubes clinking against our fancy glasses. Many times, I imagined being older, a time when I would enjoy this privilege of adulthood. That time has come. "Mom, I want a gin and tonic," I announce. Arrangements are being made for my transport to Duluth. This time I will ride in a one-engine plane, surrounded by two paramedics. We will leave in less than a week. My mom looks at me as she considers my request. What can she possibly deny me? She knows what it means and why I ask. She has watched her boy shed his childhood. She knows he has lost a lifetime.

Her friend Gudren Witrak is the smuggler. She sneaks into my room with a half-pint of gin, three six-ounce bottles of tonic, three glasses, a lime, and a knife, all packed into a mother's vast purse. The sound of breaking seals. Ice chips—not cubes—wait in our glasses. The serrated knife cuts through the lime's skin and the smell of forbidden alcohol permeates the room. I am expecting a loud transition. I am rejoining the group, but as an adult. We toast our departure, our journey home. Glasses clink in a triangle, and the adult wetness pours coolly into my mouth. I would be lying if I said it was everything I had hoped for. The moment after swallowing is nearly the same as the one before. I down the first and ask for another, hoping for the desired effect. My mom reluctantly agrees to a very light one. I drink it and wait. I look around the room, at their faces, and wonder, "Is this it?"

The moment after gin and tonics, the realization that there is not a prize behind door number one, is a moment we all share. The answer to the question "Is this it?" is, of course, yes.

We all want a simple story—I know I do. In a simple story, my paralysis and the loss of my father and sister would be the obstacles I overcome, the negatives that I turn into positives. My success would be the lessons I learned and a life of productive happiness.

In another version, the dislocation I experienced between mind and body during these months would be the injury. Yoga would eventually be the remedy. Humpty Dumpty would get put back together again, and yoga would be the glue.

My story is not simple. As I write this, I am both heartbroken and desperately in love. Living thus far has taken quite a toll. And yet, I would trade nothing. The richness and possibilities I can feel come directly from what I have experienced. I stand in awe of the transformative potential embodied by our consciousness.

This awe, however, still possesses the flavor of the moment just after gin and tonics. This fact does not weaken the drama of life. It begins it.

Part Two
Initiation

8

Into Your Arms

The day I leave Rochester to return
home to Duluth is bitterly cold. As the paramedics take me outside to load me into the plane's fuselage, they insist that I keep my
mouth covered with a blanket. It is well below zero, and I have
been inside for nearly three months. They want to protect me
from the harshness of a brutal winter. I am leaving Rochester and
still flat on my back. I have no idea what this place looks like; I
have never even seen a tree here. Is the hospital made of brick?
Does it have a courtyard? I have no idea. What I do know is that
I resent their assumption that I should not inhale the winter air.
Do they have any idea of what I have already survived? And yet,
I am also scared. I am in unknown country and going back to a
home that harbors a broken life. Maybe they do know better than
I. Maybe I do need to cover my mouth.

The wheels underneath this stretcher are cheap or too hard, or
the runway out to the plane is full of cracks. I feel every bump,
every little rock. The vibrations jiggle through my body and
tickle my ears as the rumbling sound makes my teeth grind. I

see a sharp blue sky above and watch the exhaled breath of my couriers. Time is slow and meaningful. With the plane's engine screaming against the piercing cold, I feel the weather's bite on my forehead. I move to uncover my nose. Inwardly, I am telling myself: *If I am careful and don't overdo it, I know I can breathe this invisible threat.* With the first breath, the hairs in my nose stick together. With the second, my mouth dries as it contacts a rush of freezing air. I quickly re-cover my nose. I say, "It's not so bad." I have taken a silent step toward healing.

Often I am asked what led me to eventually practice yoga. The answer is moments like these, experiences that suddenly have texture, that set deeply for no apparent reason—an unrelished hot dog, a song called "Baker Street," or stories about Australia. These are moments when somehow "more" is catalyzed, more is felt and revealed. I believe that it is the silence that makes this possible. The silence that I carried within me brought into relief these otherwise ordinary moments. I believe that the silence can deepen our perception and holds a key to our consciousness.

The moment I was rolled out to the plane matters not because I was going against the advice of the paramedics, but rather because I did not become separated from something as ordinary as the cold air. I did not overdo it, nor did I expect a miraculous result—I simply took two breaths. To see my ill-advised breaths in terms of rebelling against the medical model is to miss the point. The point is about not turning away from what is simple and straightforward, even when the surroundings are unsure. Taking two breaths can define a lifetime.

⤶

Once my mom gets me settled at the Polinsky Rehabilitation Center, she is met head-on by her broken life. She finds herself unable to plan the memorial service for my father and sister. That job has fallen to Lauren and Catherine, to the saving grace of friends. I cannot imagine what she feels as she walks through our house, as she stands next to my father's marble-top desk, or when she sees his glass piggy bank, jammed full of Depression-era fifty-cent pieces, a symbolic safety net against the farm-driven poverty of his childhood. "We'll never be poor as long as we have these coins," he would joke.

But now her partner is gone. All of my father's planning for this horrific outcome—a tidy will, a tidy estate, a formidable life insurance policy—changes little. Nothing can soften his absence. My mother is awash in a downpour of details, the crushing shift of power from the shoulders of two to the shoulders of one. Signatures and stamps and title changes and money. Clothes and closets and plans and dreams. The loss of her firstborn, an inaccessible house for her now-crippled child. Wreckage.

My mom has been avoiding this. In Rochester, the doctors, the nurses, the social workers, and even I tried to convince her to return to Duluth, to return to her house, to her life, to her other son. It would lessen the shock of it and begin the rebuilding. For my own reasons, I wanted her to go. I wanted to feel my new life on my own terms, like a kid's desire to pitch a tent in the backyard and camp out. She held firm, her reasoning sound. "I will not leave my son behind."

With this choice, my mom put caring for me between herself and her pain. I am in desperate need and young and know so little. It makes sense that she would focus on me, but she also uses me as a temporary wedge between herself and her fate. Our return to Duluth brings the outer layers of this healing maneuver under fire. She does not need to sit by my side every minute. In fact, I must learn my own initial adjustments and do so with a measure of independence. So her previous life calls her back; it is out of her control, and she is overwhelmed. Against her will, practicality forces her forward.

Not so her injured son. She can protect him from a pain she does not want to feel. My mother has decided that I will not attend the public memorial service. Instead, a small private service will be held across the hall from my hospital room in what turns out to be the mental health ward. Apparently, the mental health ward has extra meeting rooms; the rehabilitation ward does not.

My mom imagines that the strain of a public memorial service may be too much for me. But what is she protecting? My body? My heart? I suspect not. I suspect it is her body and her heart that she wants to protect but is unable to. So she protects me instead.

I am not bothered. I have never been to a memorial service or even a funeral. I do not realize what they do, how they mix collective hurt and profound cleansing. I do not know such things. I am thirteen. For me, it is just another event along the path I am surviving, like a change of body cast or sitting up in a wheelchair. If my mom organizes a special service for me, if this is how it's done, then so be it. Living within a world created by adults is nothing new, not for me, not for any child. It is how we live.

The services, both public and private, are tomorrow. Surprisingly, I am worried about what to wear. What does one wear for a trip across the hall? I have not worn clothes in over three months, and never when confined to this position. Although I am finally free of my halo cast, I am still in this wheelchair. How does one dress up? What looks good? My goal is to look strong and in some semblance of control. Worrying about appearance in the face of unwanted emotion is an avoidance technique that we all share.

When Bob, my sister's almost-fiancé, visited me in Rochester, he often wore a fantastic shirt, a kelly green turtleneck with a band of colorful racing stripes running down each arm. It looked like a ski sweater. Over and over, I told him I wanted one. Today, the day before the services, he comes to visit us in Duluth for the first time. He is bringing my copy of his shirt. The timing seems perfect. I will wear it tomorrow. As I open the package, I am slightly disappointed. It is not the same color. Mine is bright blue, but at least it is the same design. I am relieved.

I wonder if I am reaching for my sister, reaching through Bob in an unconscious expression of grief. I want to look like Bob, feel like Bob. Perhaps I imagine the shirt will protect me, connect me, help me feel through my skin what is denied through my mind.

Our meeting room is narrow and dimly lit. The lights are not standard overhead fluorescents; instead they are trying-too-hard table lamps. There are not enough of them, and the bulbs are of low wattage. The effect is to amplify the dulling assault of the orange Berber carpet that so defines the late seventies. The chairs are stiff and square and covered with plaid patterned fabric—earth-tone yellows, tans, and browns. The tables are fake wood, plastic with a grain veneer. This is where we will pray.

The day is overcast, and too many of us are stuffed into this space. There is no commanding place for the minister to stand; the result is a collective fidget. Thankfully, there is a window. Of course, it does not open, because this is the mental health ward. No air, only a view, an exit chamber for the disembodied. I stare out that window as the service begins. The scene is a Duluth hillside, rusty and decayed, displaying a tiresome and deadening winter. I feel very little, except the need to look strong, to project a pretense of realized grief.

Inwardly, I am most saddened by my appearance. I am thin and scrawny and sitting in a broken body. My plaster cast has been replaced by a removable plastic one. But I must wear it every minute of every day, even to this service. It is formed to snuggly fit my torso. It has two pieces—a front and a back—that are connected by strips of Velcro. My choices are either to wear my bright blue turtleneck underneath this body shell, a choice that would cover most of it up. Or I can wear the shirt over the body shell and look rigid and stiff, and not like a person at all. I choose the latter. In the background, I hear a blessing. It is for me and a speedy recovery. But I am disappointed . . . about my shirt.

⌒

So begins my rehabilitation. But what is it that I am rehabilitating? What is it that I am trying to "restore to a condition of good health, operation, or ability to work"? The answer to this question may seem obvious. It is not. Obviously, my back has been broken, as well as my neck and wrists. I have also been lying in bed for over three months. All of this has dramatically weakened me, but at least I am eating again and ready to begin working.

The rehabilitation model proposes that the strength in my upper body must not only be restored, but drastically increased. On top of that, the paralysis has robbed me of basic life skills. I no longer know how to dress myself, how to pee, poop, sit up from lying down, or get into a car. The focus must be to restore me to a basic level of life functionality.

This is not wrong. I must learn to do these things. The problem is that there is much more that needs to be rehabilitated. What I have actually lost in my experience of myself is an inward connection to much of my body. Below my chest has become a mental dead end—my mind has been blocked from entering. The loss of basic life skills, including my ability to walk, is simply a symptom of this mind–body dislocation.

Silence is what remains when mind becomes separated from body. My most basic unknown is how I will interact with this silence. The medical model's answer is that I won't interact with it at all. I am, instead, led to ignore it and to give up my paralyzed body as lost. Rather than working to integrate any residual silence that I might experience into who I am, I am urged to overcome it, to step over my paralysis with a courageous exertion of will. The medical model deems the air of this silence as too cold for me to breathe.

The relevance of this book turns on a simple thought. My traumatic experience of a spinal cord injury and its resulting paralysis has made more tangible a silence that exists in everyone's consciousness, a silence that can be experienced in the gap between mind and body. How we relate to this silence, how we process it, is a fundamental issue presented by our consciousness.

The solution presented by the medical model—overcoming the silence with my will—reflects a deeply embedded healing story. Thus far, human survival has been a confrontation, whether with nature, other animals, or each other. We have had to assert ourselves and become the fittest. We have taken our place at the top of the food chain. The process has not been pretty, nor has it been easy, but the ability to overcome adversity through the exertion of our will has been crucial to our survival.

Similarly, the doctors present my paralysis and its accompanying silence as things to overcome, as obstacles that I must regularly confront and then actually defeat. If I am successful in this overcoming, I will become someone to admire, someone whose story may even be inspirational.

My arms are the symbolic workhorses of this healing story. Their imagined muscle mass is proportional to the will and effort necessary to push, pull, and drag my paralyzed body through life. Their strength is what will turn the tide, what will propel me to success.

⤺

Throughout the course of my rehabilitation, I am presented with three different role models. They are the success stories of three male paraplegics. They are proven examples of the path intended for me.

Dwight is from International Falls, Minnesota. He is seventeen and has just completed his tour of duty in rehabilitation. He must have been quite a guy, leaving a wake of powerful impressions with both the physical therapists (PTs) and the nursing staff. I am told that he was an "animal" on the bench press, able to lift 190 pounds, and remember, "that's without his stomach muscles." Dwight presents an apt comparison to my situation. Although he is four years older than I am, his injury is nearly identical to mine—the fifth thoracic vertebra is broken rather than the fourth. He also lacks abdominal control.

Apparently, Dwight was injured while wildly riding his bicycle on a country road. He lost control, flew off his bike into a ditch, and hit his back against a concrete culvert. He lay there for an ungodly length of time before somebody happened by. A tough cracker is how I had imagined Dwight. He had asked to spend extra time lifting weights, did wheelies off curbs, and, by the time he left, he "had arms the size of ham hocks."

There is a problem, though. I am not that kind of athlete. True, I am very physical, but I'm not the weight-lifting type. I'm a team-sports guy, a ball lover, not a swimmer or a runner. Work and fun, that is what I respond to. Dwight, on the other hand, is a speed guy, a lover of engines. A fast talker and a fancier of trucks with roll bars, he enjoys aggressively pushing physical limits.

I do meet him some time later. He has sandy brown hair, wears a striped tank top and plain wire-rimmed glasses. He has a thick neck, and even thicker arms. We visit for a few minutes. In that time, he tells me three tales of speed and heroic endurance. He is back in the hospital after severely burning his knee. "I was ice fishing, had a few beers, and got a little too close to the woodstove. Couldn't feel a thing . . . smelled it. Imagine that, my knee melting like cheap plastic and I could only smell it," he tells me with a mixture of laughter and boasting. Dwight is an amazing guy, someone you shake your head at, smile, and hope that he stays in one piece. But for me, he does not inspire.

Meanwhile, my weight lifting is not going so well. I am told repeatedly that my arms must now do "double time for both my arms and my legs." Building in my mind is an image of my arms, a fantasy of bodybuilder arms, rippling with flex. Many people add to this image. The rehab specialists do it to motivate me; a male nurse tells me that "chicks are going to dig it," and with approving eyes, my friends and family beam, "Wow, those arms are going to be huge." In fact, this healing story is still projected at me some twenty-five years later, now mostly by strangers. They see me pushing my wheelchair up a hill or putting it in my car and want to say something, empower me somehow, encourage the will they imagine it takes to overcome a disability. From the sidewalk, they might give me a thumbs-up, maybe even yell "Rock on." Of course, the unspoken subtext of this cultural healing story is "You may not have legs, but wow, do you have arms."

During my workouts in rehab, however, I drift out the window, not into my arms. I sit at the arm pulleys intending to do my five sets of twelve. Instead, time stretches out. I watch the flurry of activity in front of me. The rehab gym is full of people: standing people, walking people, sitting people, unable-to-talk people. Most of them are older, their dysfunction brought on by age. I am in between, too old for pediatric rehabilitation and definitely the lone boy beginning puberty. As I watch this scene, I set it against the view out the large, south-facing windows. My eyes are out of focus and gazing into the gray sky. This scene repeats over and over, day after day. I am not making the progress they would like, but through silence I continue to smile. I am aging much too quickly.

They keep changing my physical therapist. I suspect that they want to jump-start my progress, find a PT for whom I will work harder. I am gaining skills but at a slow pace, being just as happy to socialize with the therapists as I am to work. I like knowing about them and their lives. I like the feeling of them liking me, but not the feeling of my muscles against their weights. Something feels intuitively wrong about how I am being told to work. I am to press aggressiveness through my upper body: push, pull, jerk, and get the job done. But hasn't enough of that energy already traveled through me? I am tired of bouncing and crashing and crawling back to center. I am willing to work, but let it be smooth, balanced, and even, like shooting a perfect free throw. This silence demands grace, not rupture.

Enter Rick, their ace in the hole, the PT who delivered Dwight to his heroic stature. Rick wears rimless octagonal glasses and hiking boots, has longish hair, and is the first vegetarian I have ever met. What he eats for lunch fascinates me. I am from a meat-and-potatoes family, and he strikes me as a quasi-alien. It turns out that his lunches aren't that interesting—bits and pieces that add up to a meal: nuts and raisins, carrots and celery, and a peanut-butter-and-jelly sandwich. It seems normal enough, but I keep a suspicious eye on his paper sack, waiting to view the secret of what those people really eat.

Rick is sharp with my ways of procrastination. His voice is impatient when we are working. Joking is not an option. He is the first male therapist I have had, and his manner is different. He does not comment on my soft eyes or my long eyelashes. He has no interest in finding the hurting young child adrift in the silence. He challenges me to step up and "be a man."

We are on an elevated, eight-by-eight-foot brown mat. In the last few days, I have just begun to make sliding board transfers. I direct my wheelchair alongside the mat; it is about four inches lower than my seat. I put one end of the board under my leg and the other on the destination. Lifting my body as best I can, I begin the slide downward. Sliding board transfers are the first and, for some, the only way to move in and out of a wheelchair. Eventually, with increased strength and a better sense of balance, no board is needed—one just hoists the body from one place to another. It is a long way off for me. Learning how to lift my legs onto the mat is also a challenge—a surprisingly delicate balance when living in a body without adequate sensors. But this, too, I am beginning to master.

Once on the mat, I feel like an exposed fish. There is no order to movement, just the stuck feeling of being contained within a strange body and under the heavy press of gravity. As I lie flat on my back, we work on sitting up from a lying-down position. I have already learned one technique. I roll onto my side, a formidable task in itself, which usually requires that I grab the side of the mat, then press down through my elbow and move onto my forearm. My other hand then pushes into the mat and, if the planets are aligned just right, I raise myself into a sitting position. But this method is not adequate for Rick—it has too many movements and takes too much time. There is a more direct way. While lying flat on my back, I am to force my elbows underneath me, then rock from side to side until enough momentum is created to make the space for one arm and elbow to lock straight. This, in turn, creates the space to lock the other arm straight. Once both hands are pressing into the mat, I am to rock back and forth and lift into an upright position. It is a difficult maneuver that takes much more strength and is particularly hard on the muscles that attach to my shoulder blades.

Not only am I unable to make the initial lift onto my elbows, I cannot get from there to an upright position. I am not aggressive enough and, by implication, not man enough. We have been working on it for days to no avail. We are both frustrated. After yet another failure, I gripe, "Why can't I just do it the other way?" Rick slams his hand on the mat, slides off, and says in a disgusted tone, "Dwight could do it, but fine, if you want to live like a quadriplegic all your life, go ahead."

Apparently, quadriplegics do things one way and paraplegics another. Rick has mixed shame into my sense of failure. Is he miffed because my life will be adversely affected by an inability to aggressively sit up? Or is he tweaked because he hasn't gotten the results he wanted? I wonder whose failure he is ashamed of. I am too young for these thoughts and instead pass deeper into silence.

Even this morning, all these years later, I was practicing yoga and was still able to feel Rick's biting words. Now, I am strong enough to sit up in any way I want and more supple within my body than I ever imagined possible. I tried sitting up the aggressive way and then the "quadriplegic" way. The difference is that the latter is much more graceful.

Once again, I am lying on the mat, but now I am creating a little stir. For the last couple of hours, groups of physical therapists, including Rick, are standing in little huddles and talking

quietly about me. Excitement hangs in the air. Beginning yesterday, there has been movement in my left foot—I seem to be able
to flex it slightly back toward my face. Taken by itself, this is not
such a big deal. Many spinal cord injuries create spasticity, a random firing of muscle fibers producing involuntary movement.
But this movement appears to be different. It looks like I am con-
trolling it, hence the whispering. They are whispering because they
worry that my hopes will suddenly reverse, that I will become
convinced that I am the lucky one, the one who will walk again.
And what if it is a false alarm? Then my hopes will be dashed,
acceptance will have to be relearned, all amounting to lost time.

I am examined independently by three different PTs. They ask
me to move my foot. I move it. Mostly, I'm having fun; the
heightened attention is pleasing. I feel like I have found twenty
dollars in a pair of discarded pants. My mind is not really racing
ahead; it all feels too unreal, more like a happy dream. But their
secrecy, their obvious attempt not to include me, gets me wondering, "Hey, maybe something really is up!" The possibility
makes me feel proud. "See, there is too some life down there in
those legs."

Amidst the hubbub, a PT student takes her turn with me.
Laurie is overtly sweet, breathy, well intentioned, and has dark
brown Farrah Fawcett hair. A cheerleader in high school, she will
finish her degree in the allotted time and then promptly marry
her sweetheart, the gorgeous guy who just happened to be the
captain of the hockey team. She notices something the others
have missed. When I try to move my foot, both my neck and
latissimus dorsi (middle side back) muscles flex. She determines

that I am creating the groundbreaking movement with my upper body. In short, she decides that I have been cheating. The others agree. As quickly as the excitement arose, it disappears. Huddles break up, whispering stops, and it is back to the matters at hand. In fact, they want me to forget the whole incident.

"Matt, you need to stop thinking about this, start thinking about your arms again," the voice commands. "What matters most for you now is working on practical tasks and building arm strength."

"But what about moving my foot?"

"That doesn't matter. It doesn't mean anything. Nothing has changed. You just devised a clever way to make it look otherwise. You tricked us."

"I wasn't trying to trick anyone. It just seemed like I could move my foot."

"I know, but don't hold on to that. It has no neurological implications. Your severed spinal cord is not spontaneously reconnecting. You're still completely paralyzed. The faster you accept that and move on, the better."

I feel humiliated, silly that I even attempted to move my foot. I remember my forgotten phantom feelings. Once again, I feel oddly ashamed. "Sorry, I don't mean to be a bother," I want to call out, to save face. "I wasn't trying to escape my life . . . I just thought . . . I'm sorry . . . I'll try to do better."

That boy has sting on his face. They have set yet another healing story, a pivotal one. It is the practical complement to the story
about the phantom feelings. The doctors have already convinced
me that any sensation that I might hear within my paralyzed body
isn't real; that it doesn't, in fact, exist. Now, the PTs set forth a
reality picture that values only one kind of reconnection with my
paralyzed body, namely one that travels physiologically through
my spinal cord. Anything short of that I must leave behind. I must
move willfully into my arms and forward with a body that is
barely mine.

There is another way forward, however. A spinal cord injury is
experienced fundamentally as a mind-body injury. Is reversing
the damage to my spinal cord the only holy grail here, the only
potential source of mind-body integration?

My injury is experienced inwardly as a separation between
mind and body. This makes reconnecting my mind to my body
essential to my healing process. This, in turn, makes it imperative
that I can conceive of ways to do so. I accept that I will never
walk again. But the ability to voluntarily move my paralyzed legs
is not the only measure of success. There are others. For starters,
it is important for me to experience any kind of connection to my
paralyzed body that I can.

Was it healing when I was moving my foot even though I was
"cheating"? Yes, yes, yes. Was it a beginning step in my process of
mind-body reintegration? Yes, yes, yes. Anything I do to reconnect my presence to my paralyzed body is a form of healing. So
what if I used my back and neck muscles to move my foot? I was
making a connection to my body below the point of my injury. It

was groundbreaking. I was moving through the silence of my paralysis and toward my body.

This marked the beginning of perhaps my most important realization—that there is healing other than healing to walk again. I do not mean simply that more than physical healing is possible, for example, additional psychological and emotional healing. I mean that healing is still possible for my mind-body relationship, and it doesn't mean that I will walk again. Unfortunately, I do not fully grasp this until I begin to practice yoga many years later. In the meantime, that thirteen-year-old boy was stuck believing that the damage to his spinal cord was irreversible. More important, he believed that reversing it was his only healing option. In such a case, where could his healing go? "Into your arms," the voices boom.

9

Wheels, Not Legs

They say a frog thrown into boiling water will jump out. But a frog set in cold water brought slowly to a boil will remain until it is too late. The long-term effect of my rehabilitation was like entering a slow boil. Over time, I became a shell of myself. I was able to maintain a smile pointed outward to gather the world's approval, but inwardly, I was turning gray and creeping dangerously close to dissolution. Thankfully, I am a lucky frog and was able to jump out.

The second of my potential role models is shuffled through my thirteen-year-old awareness. Dennis is an amazing guy. He owns a business, is an active citizen within his community, and even serves on his town council. He is a friend of a friend of my father. I can tell my mom is excited for me to meet him. This is the person she envisions as a role model. She wants me to see someone living an active life, a normal guy who just happens to be a paraplegic.

Dennis is married, has curly brown hair and a catchy smile. *Married* catches my ear, as I am afraid that this is no longer possible for me.

"Were you married before or after?" I ask.

"Before . . . and had two kids." My heart sinks a little. But I am trying to see as much as I can in Dennis. I want to please my mom.

"Did she have trouble adjusting—your wife, I mean?" I am still looking for my angle.

"Why would she? I'm still the same guy." I hesitate as I wonder if what he says is true. "She's been great, really been there for me. Wasn't always easy, but we managed just fine."

I am feeling uplifted, like something about my life ahead can be normal. I want him to talk about little things, like speaking at a public meeting or eating at a restaurant. I do not know how to ask such questions or even that I want to know such things. But I do want something, an intangible. I want him to tell me that I will have a place in the world.

The conversation lags as I struggle to get what I need. Dennis reaches into his bag and pulls out a series of pictures. It is not joy on his face; it is stern satisfaction, his accomplishment, his proof. Apparently, Dennis was quite a deer hunter before his accident. He still is. He tells me a story about last year's hunt, about killing, gutting, and dragging a deer from the woods without anyone's help. He has the pictures to prove it. There is one qualification though. "I did use an ATV four-wheeler," he laughs as he pretends that this might tarnish his achievement. As I am playing along, I try to laugh with him. "But at least I hooked the chains up by myself." His sentence hangs in the air because our laughter was false. Each time I try to bring the conversation somewhere else, he inevitably swings it back to his trophy. "I didn't go this year, got too busy. But next year, you can bet . . ."

His hunting story is so dominant that it pretty much ends the visit. I close my eyes and try to absorb his tale in the spirit it was offered. He is giving me a gift, a marker, proof that his continuity has remained. That mine will, too. With enough determination— a four-wheeler notwithstanding—anything is possible. His healing story has been earned through his will.

I am confused by his visit, saddened. I am old enough to think that he has missed the point, that he misplaces his accomplishments. His community-oriented life proves its own worth, not the deer he drags from the woods. And yet, fifteen years later, I will make my version of this mistake. My body will pay the price.

The third role model takes the medical model's healing vision a step deeper. Steve is the older brother of Sheila, my junior high school crush. She ends up being my girlfriend for much of the eighth and ninth grades. Steve is famous within the Duluth rehab community. He was injured when he was sixteen, while swimming in the nearby Lester River. As I understand it, his buddy jumped off a bridge and landed on Steve's back. He too is injured at about the fourth thoracic vertebra. Quite an athlete and swimmer before his accident, Steve excelled afterward, winning multiple gold medals at the worldwide Paralympics.

I too am quite an athlete. The feeling of playing sports is probably the purest love I have ever experienced. Even now, all these years later, I still have dreams in which I make some sort of recovery, just enough to strap it on and grace the basketball court or the baseball diamond. Never at 100 percent, there is always some vestige of waking life—a limp, an inability to run at full speed, a sore back, something—but I am out there making the best of it. Usually, I am unable to sustain the pace of the game and the dream slowly fades. Not painfully, just fades.

Upon reaching rehab in Duluth, I am barraged by stories of wheelchair athletics, what's out there, what's possible. The intent is to soften my loss by showing me what I can still do, what athletic expression is still available to me. If I can get back on the horse, so to speak, then I can prove that my disability has not kept me down, has not changed me too much.

Steve is the wildly successful embodiment of this healing vision. His arms are the news. "Swimming is a fabulous way to strengthen the upper body," I am told. My imagination cannot really envision how a paralyzed body swims, but no matter. I am anxious to meet Steve, even nervous. It's not that I am excited by wheelchair sports. My heart is too sore to truly go there. But I am curious on a couple of levels. First and foremost, I want to see those arms, how they ripple, how they look in clothes. Will they stand out? Will their strength be tangibly felt? I want to know.

My other curiosity, one I cannot really articulate, is what a stellar wheelchair athlete will look like. Will something stick out about Steve, something that marks him as an exceptional athlete? As he comes around the corner, he is wearing a jacket. I am disappointed. How am I going to see those pipes? He has brown hair, quite a thick mustache, and serious eyes. He is about twice my age, and his upper body seems to dwarf the back of his wheelchair's seat. *There is wonder hidden under that jacket,* I think to myself, but we talk about wheelchairs. His is so different from the hospital loaner I am using—lower, more compact, seemingly contoured around his body. This isn't far from the case. The cutting-edge modification done for sporty wheelchairs is called cambering the axles. This angles the wheels so the space between them is wider at the ground than it is at the top. It also slightly reduces the width of the seat back. So Steve's torso is, literally, bulging out of his chair.

"Why is your chair like that?" I ask.

"You mean the wheels? Well, there are a couple of reasons. The wider wheel base on the bottom saves the hands. Going through a narrow doorway, the bottom hits, not the top."

"You're kidding. I never would have thought of that."

"You're new at this. The cambering also makes the chair more snug, makes you able to change direction with only your torso; it makes the chair more responsive." I am getting an education. I know this is supposed to be cool. "The axles are also moved forward to make the chair extra tippy."

"Why?"

"That way you can pop a wheelie just by leaning back." He

sees the lost look in my eyes. "When you come to a curb, you don't have to break your momentum by touching the wheels; you can just pop the front wheels up and get over." This explanation means nothing to me. He smiles and nods, "You'll see." After a pause, he says, "Having the axles forward also makes a tighter turning radius. It helps getting out of tight spots. You'll have a few of those." He laughs again and shows me by maneuvering around my hospital room. "Last but not least, having the back wheels moved forward creates better pushing power. You can grab farther back on the wheels, get a longer push." He demonstrates by leaning forward and taking an imaginary stroke.

"It looks like you're sitting at an angle, with your butt lower than your knees," I say.

"Good eye. You're catching on. This also helps pushing power. In order to get the leverage for a good push, you need to get your head and shoulders out over your legs. Sitting on a slant forces you to lean forward." Again, he demonstrates. His body position brings to mind a rocket.

We move out to the hall and he shows me how well his chair works by zipping around. He is so adept; his chair glides with fluid speed like a wave beginning to break. Body and chair moving as one, they have merged. His legs overruled by wheels, his upper body leads his presence, while his new, circular limbs distribute his strength. He and I are so very different.

We move back into my hospital room. I catch a break. Apparently hot from wheeling around, Steve removes his leather jacket. There they are: the arms I have been waiting for. They do not disappoint. They have amazing bulk, not rippling but shapely, even when not flexed. I want to see them at full engagement and am tempted to ask him to imitate a bodybuilder. Thankfully, I feel too silly. I do notice a tattoo on the outside of his right arm. Back in the late seventies, tattoos are still the domain of motorcycle gangs, at least to a thirteen-year-old. *I bet he parties,* I think to myself. Regardless, the tattoo gives me an excuse to stare at his arms.

The visit finishes up. Steve puts on his jacket, covers those arms, and wheels off. Moving quickly down the hall, he cuts even more crisply around the corner as rubber pivots against tiled floor. I am left in a wake of confidence and cool. As my thoughts linger, it feels like the visit will simply rewind and begin again, as if I am watching a repeating film clip.

Back in my room, I am trying to reconfigure myself in light of what I have seen. *So this is how it will be.* I am simultaneously relieved and unnerved. With more experience and a better wheelchair, I won't always feel so awkward, so out of place. Eventually, I will feel like I am sitting *in* a wheelchair, not *on* one, that balance and focus will lead my movement, not the lumbering feeling of disconnection. But I am also unnerved by Steve's presence. Losing boundary between myself and my wheelchair, becoming the speed of wheels and arms—is this the way forward?

Something in me resists. I love the feeling of my body. I always have, that's why I have loved playing sports. The feeling of a baseball making quintessential contact with a bat, the hands gaining a privileged glimpse into a sudden elasticity of wood. The sound of a golf ball bursting forth from the driver's sweet spot, the effortless soaring of what ensues. But a basketball shot, that's even more serious. Not pure joy, there is more intent, a conscious collapsing of hoop, ball, and distance, all mediated by feeling. The feeling of the ball rotating off the fingertips like a lingering touch, the uncorking spring in legs and feet that fuel the ball's rainbow arc, the satisfying sound of the ball cutting through the net. Sensual beauty disguised as competition.

Steve shows me more than how a wheelchair athlete looks or what magnificent pipes look like draped under bikers' leather. He also shows me the natural consequence of a compensating healing vision, one that relies so heavily upon his arms. My legs will be traded for the technology of wheelchairs. I am being led to leave my paralyzed body behind and willfully engage the rest, to merge with my wheelchair and not look back.

Steve is only a messenger. In truth, what makes me uneasy has nothing to do with him and everything to do with me, with who I am, and who I want to be. As I consider the healing story that Steve embodies, my love of my body recoils and falls into invisible grass. It moves off to the side and waits. A lucky frog.

In some ways, everyone faces a similar choice about his or her body. As I strap myself behind the wheel of my car, in a virtual cockpit of lights and gadgets, as I move my consciousness into yet another technology screen—whether television, computer, or cell phone—I know that I am disconnecting from my body. When I watch relatively healthy people ride the moving sidewalks in air-port terminals or take an elevator up a single floor, I wonder about these choices. When I trade the feeling of warm water run-ning over my hands for the convenience of a dishwasher, I know that I am losing something.

These are not mistakes or moral failings. They are simply choices. They are choices we make that define how we interact with our bodies, and they shape our consciousness. If I had chosen to embrace the speed of my wheelchair and become a successful wheelchair athlete, you would not have judged me to be morally lacking. In fact, you might have admired my determination. These choices do not make us good or bad people. But they do determine the connection we experience to our bodies.

The Industrial Revolution and Information Age have had an unintended consequence—they have moved us farther away from our bodies. This is not a necessary consequence, however. I am not saying that we should spurn technology. That's as silly as say-ing that I should have refused to use a wheelchair. I can use my wheelchair and still keep a vibrant connection to my whole body. It does mean, though, that I must make the process of integration with my paralyzed body more conscious, more focused. As a paraplegic, I can no longer rely on the normal course of my daily life to ensure a healthy connection between my mind and my body. The same is true for all of us.

∽

It is nearing the time when I will leave the hospital and live at home. Now I am even able to sit in my wheelchair without my body brace. So tiring, so naked this feels, but I am finally winning, finally becoming a body free of medical props. After just two hours of this sitting, however, I must sleep, not just because I am simply tired, but because I feel boneless, shapeless, without clear definition. Instability along the spine is like stepping off a three-inch curb and having it turn out to be a six-inch drop. It is not the pain of your surprised knee joint as it receives the pavement. It is the groundless feeling of reaching for the pavement while in descent. But I am healing; somehow, my body is healing. Each day, the lost reference within my back becomes more found. I am regaining autonomous shape, the sturdy, upright feeling that distinguishes your skin from the world around it. As my shoulders, head, and neck regain their confidence, my view is recovering its platform.

My mom and I have two final consultations with my doctors. The first one is with my orthopedist. He is the man who was my sister's godfather and also arranged for my transfer from the hospital in Des Moines to the Mayo Clinic. My mom and I trust him completely.

The meeting is in a hallway. It is brief and to the point. He flicks my most recent back x-ray into the clip that holds the black-and-white transparency over a fluorescent wall light. The warbling sound of the bending x-ray fills my head. Dr. Van Pufflen's expression is austere, his upper lip pulled tightly across his teeth. He is my doctor, but he is also sad.

"Matt, Paula, let me get you referenced here." His finger runs across the picture. "As you can see, these are the Harrington rods." I cannot believe how literal they look—parallel columns with interlocking nuts, bolts, and hooks—easily something that could have been purchased at a hardware store. "See how the x-ray shows there is no space between the vertebrae here?" Now, a pointing pen slides over the image of my spine. "This is where you have been fused. It all looks to be holding together wonderfully. That's the good news." He pauses and catches both of our gazes. "It's below this point that's of concern. Well, not concern. It was expected, but I was hoping you'd get lucky. But see how your spine is beginning to curve." The pen travels to the vertebrae just below the rods. My stare is fixed; my breathing is shallow but peaceful. I am used to getting bad news. "We don't know where that curving process will stop."

He goes on to explain that my back is forming what is called *traumatically acquired scoliosis*. The surgeons at the Mayo Clinic had opted not to fuse my entire spine. Their hope was that the extra rigid support would not be needed. But because my upper back is so stabilized and I lack any abdominal control, there is no resistance to hold my curving middle spine in check.

My mom is silent. She is waiting for his guidance. Finally, I ask, "What can we do?"

"For now, nothing. We have to wait and see. We'll monitor it on a yearly basis."

"And if it continues?" my mom asks.

"If it gets beyond a certain point, Matt will have the rest of his back fused." I am not reacting; unconsciously, my mind shifts to survival.

"What does that mean? What kind of recovery period?" my tone flatly demands.

"Let's not go there. It may not happen." He sees that my hard stare will not release him. "After the surgery, a month or more in bed, some time in a body cast, and then about six months in a brace similar to the one you are wearing now." My mom looks at me; she knows my heart is breaking. I am still looking for a way out.

"There must be something we can do," my voice implores.

He clears his throat. "There's nothing. We have to let nature take its course . . . see where your spine lands. It's out of our hands." As my attempt at anger gives way to an onrush of silence, I feel sleepy.

This is another bad healing story. I have been made subject to my back, to a passive hope that it won't curve any more. I leave that meeting disheartened. The force of the blow to my upper back is continuing its wayward dance. The first wave registered in an instant and shredded my spinal integrity. This second wave— an echoing of sorts—extends my breaking, slowly, over time. Never free of its grip, my only option is to wait for it to get worse. I feel an accelerated glimpse into death, into a dissipation of form. I feel like I am flying apart, like I did on the Foster frame in the intensive care unit. And yet, I find myself wheeling down a cor- ridor to an elevator, to push a button, to return to my temporary home, to where I will push another button that raises and lowers the height of my bed.

Our second consultation is with Dr. Goff, my rehabilitation doctor. He has recently finished his residency at the Mayo Clinic. He comes highly recommended by my previous rehab doctor, the one from the tundra I imagine as Iceland. He is soft-spoken and avoids eye contact. He is left-handed and curls his forearm and wrist as he writes, as if protecting something precious. He always looks like he just woke up from a nap, his wavy hair in disarray. The meeting is in his office, a room just off the physical therapy gym. This morning he looks particularly disheveled. His tone is factual as he lays out my prognosis during a sweeping monologue.

"Living with a spinal cord injury is hard work." He forces a glance upward at us and then returns to his downward gaze. "Of course, Matt will never walk again, but you already know that. His best bet is using a wheelchair, as he is not a viable candidate for long-legged braces." My mom and I are both surprised. There has been virtually no talk of this option. I figure he must be covering all the bases, regardless of the particular patient. "Obviously, a central issue confronting a paraplegic is bladder and bowel management. I recommend that Matt continue using a Uro Sheath—an external catheter. Our attempts at training his bladder to follow a structured emptying pattern have for the most part failed. This is not a surprising result, and his bladder seems to empty well enough on its own. Many of our patients find the Uro Sheath the most practical, hassle-free option anyway. As far as

Matt's bowels are concerned, that is pretty much up to you. Suppositories or digital stimulation, it's your choice."

I am getting irritated. I want something new and important from this meeting, not a rehashing of what I already know. "Spasticity. Matt does suffer some from this. We could medicate, usually with Valium, but he has made it clear that he wants to keep his mind as sharp as possible." I smile faintly with some pride; I have shown some mettle. "If the spasticity ever becomes too burdensome, however, then come back and see me. Sexual intercourse. The ability for a paraplegic to experience an erection varies from case to case. You'll have to wait and see." I smile because I already know this is not a problem for me. "Children. The likelihood that Matt will ever biologically father a child is slim to none. This is true for two reasons. First, the sperm tends to be of lower quality. We think this is because the temperature in the reproductive system is higher than normal due to sitting all the time." He waits for comments. I have none. I didn't know the details, but I knew the result. The silence has already helped me accept what I am too young to want. He continues, "Second, if the patient is capable of ejaculation at all, it is usually what we call *retrograde ejaculation*. This means that the sperm travels not outward through the penis but back into the bladder."

"Why?" I ask.

"We don't know." Dr. Goff forces another look up to acknowledge ignorance and moves on. "The most troublesome long-term issue facing spinal cord injuries is urinary tract infections. There is really no way around this. Your bladder, Matt, just doesn't empty as well or as often as the average person's. This means it is

a wet, dark, warm place—a breeding ground for bacteria. I recommend that he take a half-dose of antibiotic each day."

"For the rest of my life?" I blurt out.

"I'm afraid so. This is the best option against what is a potentially serious problem. The leading cause of death among spinal
cord injuries is kidney failure, and there is a direct correlation
between frequent bladder infections and kidney trouble. In fact,
Matt is a likely candidate for dialysis later in life." This hospital
has recently opened a dialysis unit. A nurse took me to see it, but
I hadn't known why. My face is beginning to sting. "Another big
problem area is skin breakdown. Matt has already experienced a
host of pressure sores. This is somewhat worrisome. You see, each
time the skin breaks down, it regenerates only about 70 percent of
its previous resilience—the more it breaks down, the more likely
it is to break down. Matt will have to watch this closely. A major
pressure sore is both costly and time-consuming, usually weeks in
the hospital. We have taught him about constant weight shifts
while sitting and have given him two mirrors so he can inspect
the skin on his butt each and every day." The word *butt* sounds so
funny coming out of Dr. Goff's mouth—an off-balance attempt
to display comfort with bodies and people and informing patients
of their bleak futures. I can't tell if his factual approach is a device
to protect a big heart or if his shyness hides a deep-seated disin-
terest in the actual lives of others. What I do know is that I am
growing tired of his voice, his flat intonation, and his brown half-
boots that zip on the inside of each ankle. "Another problem Matt
faces is hyperdysreflexia . . ."

I am no longer listening. My mom looks frozen—legs crossed,

smile pasted on, and breathless. I know this look. She has hit a wall; her lack of movement and smiling politeness betray that she is frantic. This is not the life she wants for her youngest son. I, on the other hand, am looking for a way to break the drone of what we have heard, for a way to bring movement back to my mom's eyes. As Dr. Goff finishes up, I ask through a playful smile, "So what's the good news?" The surprised look on his face and rush to answer mean that he thinks I actually want an answer.

"Well, Matt . . . if you follow the programs of maintenance we have taught you, if you are vigilant about your health and upkeep, you can expect a relatively normal life."

Yippee.

The disintegration of body. We are all living a death sentence of sorts, and it is delivered to us through the disintegration of our bodies. In some ways, I was lucky to be exposed to this truth so early. If the arc of life is drawn as a bell curve, then at thirteen I received this news on the upslope. So much lay before me—the natural momentum of my life force was still strongly forward. This was not a decision that required effort. It was an energetic fact.

Seeking begins when the options presented are unacceptable. The path before me included a troubled mind-body relationship and dwindling prospects of health. At thirteen, these truths were not obstacles to confront. They were part of the air that I was breathing. If I was going to live, I needed to *live* the mind-body relationship my life had dealt me. My arm strength didn't have to overcome it. Unfortunately, this would take years for me to realize.

Even now, I can still hear myself answering my father during that summer between third and fourth grades. Can I control accidents . . . the course of my life . . . my disintegration? Not exactly, but I can *live* the experience I actually have. Seeking means believing in one's experience. I think he would have liked this answer.

What this implies for my experience of rehabilitation is something else again.

the shaw of repeated meam

10

Broken Again

Imagine walking from a well-lit room into a dark one. Imagine the darkness as a visual expression of silence. My rehabilitation made a mistake with the silence by focusing on the absence of light. It too quickly accepted the loss and taught me to willfully strike out against the darkness. It told me to move faster rather than slower, push harder rather than softer. It guided me to compensate for what I could not see.

Another course of action, however, is patience. Stop moving, wait for the eyes to adjust, allow for stillness, and then see what's possible. Although full-fledged vision does not return, usually there is enough light to find one's way across the room. After a while, the moon may come out, sounds might gain texture, and the world might reveal itself once again, only darker.

I was convinced to accept a complete loss of light. First, the doctors replaced the flesh and bones of my legs and feet with stories of phantoms and ghosts. Next, the physical therapists guided me to believe that the only meaningful connection to my paralyzed body was through a regenerating spinal cord. Against this backdrop, compensation was offered. My arms and my wheels, fueled by a compensating will, were to carry me through my life. My efforts would aim to prove that the room's darkness didn't matter at all. I would overcome it and become as effective as if the light were still on.

But what if I really wanted to be whole? If I wanted to work *with* the darkness rather than *against* it? Such questions were beyond the range of my rehabilitation. My initial attempts to feel my whole body were seen as an impossible hope to walk again. The only other option presented to me was total darkness—my paralyzed body as lost. This was the mistake. When silence is perceived strictly as loss, it can become deadening, even self-destructive. In my case, my paralyzed body became a static weight, an antithesis to living presence.

This view of silence lends itself to a familiar story. We love the notion of overcoming adversity, of succeeding in the face of imminent and probable failure. Short of that, we admire those who refuse to fall without a fight. We are a willful culture and define our heroes accordingly. We strive for victory over the darkness of the room.

But what if the darkness (the silence) is a fundamental part of us, of our consciousness? How do we *overcome* an essential aspect of what we are? For me, as we shall see, working against the silence deadened my sense of living and accelerated a negative sense of death.

Eventually, I reached a boiling point. But the lucky frog in me refused to trade my lower body for the speed of will and wheels. When I resisted this particular healing story, when I instead actively explored the silence, a different world appeared, one with greater depth and potential.

⌣

My first day home from the hospital is the first day of June 1979, some six months after the accident. Although I will continue physical therapy as an outpatient through the fall, it feels good to be home. I will be living in our sunroom.

The space is ten feet by ten feet, with windows all around and a dark stone floor. While I was growing up, the sunroom offered me my first measure of independence during my Saturday morning ritual. I would wake up, grab a quilt, get a bowl of Cap'n Crunch, and buckle in for a journey through cartoon heaven—*Pink Panther*, *Scooby-Doo*, Looney Tunes, and, of course, *Jonny Quest*. The entrance to this room, about seven feet wide, served as the goal crease for Nerf hockey, the goal line for "goal-line stand" football, and generally a boundary between imagined worlds.

Now it is the opening to both my bedroom and my bathroom. My bed is against the wall where our black-and-white TV was— my dad had refused to follow our culture into color—and a commode is wheeled in when I need to empty my bowels. The shower is upstairs, and my brother is the designated courier of my body. He is eighteen and working summer nights at a grocery distribution warehouse until four in the morning. My mom rustles him out of bed at nine, and in an exhausted trance, he carries me up the winding stairs, sets me on a chair, turns on the shower, and collapses back into bed, only to reverse the process in fifteen minutes. I try not to shower very often.

By mid-August, an addition to our house will be complete. We are converting our garage into a bedroom, adding a bathroom with a wheel-in shower, a side entryway, and a new, two-car garage. I will have what feels like my own wing of the house.

For the next year, my mother and brother fight like cats and dogs. Each wants what the other cannot give. My mom wants another adult, someone to share responsibilities, decisions, concerns—some level of companionship in what is now a makeshift family. My brother is ready to break away. He aches for a normal transition away from parental control and into independence. Just last summer, he was traveling across Europe with his intensive history and literature class. He drank his first hard cider, had a hot romance with a girl abroad, and came back on top of the world. Upon his return, our family, minus Laura, met him in New York and toured prospective colleges: Harvard, Yale, Princeton, Dartmouth, Brown, the University of Michigan, and Northwestern. As a top student, James could have gone wherever he pleased.

But now, my mom is insisting that he go to school in Duluth. "We need to stick together right now. Too much has happened." Frankly, I am relieved. Not having my brother around is unimaginable. He also knows this, knows that his obligation is to us. But this means he must stand by and watch as his life continues to break. Like all of us, he is trying to heal, searching for continuity, a way to recognize and connect who he was before the accident with who he is after. On each day that he goes to the wrong school, he is made to look squarely into the face of his damaged life. Thwarted, frustrated, and angry, he grinds through his first year at the University of Minnesota in Duluth. He and my mom will compromise. James will transfer to the University of Minnesota, Twin Cities, the following year; 150 miles seems like a manageable distance for our family to absorb.

Still, my mother and brother continue to fight. My brother needs attention, some sort of acknowledgment that he too has suffered. People can more readily relate to a mother who has lost her husband and firstborn child; and they can plainly see my physical damage. Not so the ruptured world of the older, walking brother. When he reaches out to our mom, he sees only that she is consumed with helping me. In some ways, he is still alone in our house and we are still in Rochester. He develops a do–it–on–his–own streak and is willful enough to carry himself forward. He moves through college and law school and successfully builds his own law firm. But the cost has been high. He too has poured much of his hurt into the silence.

My mom settles into a widow's life. In the first few years, she gets her master's in art and has multiple marriage proposals. Twice she gets pretty serious, only to find the suitors lacking. When I ask her for her thoughts in retrospect, she says, "They just weren't interesting enough. Your father so fascinated me." The result is a woman who lives with three animals, continues to paint, loves her people, and quietly reads while listening to classical music.

Through it all, we remain a close-knit family. Never quite getting what we want from each other, we continue to eat food around tables, are deeply committed to each other's well-being, and have a tendency to dwell on the past. We don't fixate on the good ole days before the accident, but rather speculate about the relationships we don't get to have, about the mystery of what becomes of people who have died. We are still processing twenty-five years later. I imagine we always will.

I returned to Ordean Junior High School during that same year, in September 1979, more than nine months after the car accident. I was passed on to eighth grade even though I had missed three-quarters of seventh grade. I needed to stay with my friends, and the school district reluctantly agreed. I was a smart kid and could make up for lost time. It wasn't quite that easy. Six months of school is a lot to miss—it took about a year for me to truly catch up.

I had the most amazing friends—Roger, Mark, Tom, John, Sheila, Annelise, Kerri, and others. We picked up right where we left off. Yes, things were different. Yes, I rolled to destinations rather than walked, and peed into a bag attached to my leg rather than into a toilet, but my friends took me everywhere. We traveled in a pack, my friends taking turns pushing me up the steep hills of Duluth and then fighting to catch a ride standing on the back of my wheelchair while rolling down them. We went to movies, listened to music, talked, and had water fights. Girls sat on my lap, and girls and boys even kissed each other on occasion.

With a web of close friends, returning to the social side of school was easier than I expected. I had two advantages. My disability did not disfigure me. At first glance, I looked like an average kid who just happened to be sitting in a wheelchair. This made my reimmersion into the greater student population much easier. Besides bumping into the heels of kids standing in the hallways, I wasn't scary. For the most part, I didn't make people feel uncomfortable.

The other advantage I had was a celebrity status of sorts. Although I was in seventh grade for less than three months, I had made a lot of friends. I had also been elected to the student council and had been the only seventh grader on both the varsity softball and basketball teams. My peers were ready and waiting for the return of the kid who was in that "terrible car accident."

Returning to the physical side of school was not so easy. My school was on three floors, and there was no elevator. My wheelchair and I would get tipped back into a wheelie and bumped up or down a flight of stairs one step at a time. Two of my friends—Roger and John—took turns between classes teaming with a female aid to perform the lifting duties. Ironically, both my junior and senior high schools got elevators within the first few years after I left.

In the classroom, it didn't get much better. None of the combination chair/desks worked for a kid in a wheelchair. The school administration found two desks that I could wheel under and have a writing surface. I picked the two classes in which I needed them the most—algebra and English. Situated in the front corner of each room, I sat behind my special desk and tried not to feel conspicuous. In the other classes, I wrote on my lap.

The bathrooms were not at all wheelchair accessible. This just compounded my most stressful problem—managing my bladder and bowels. I was still new at being a paraplegic and had not found my body's new rhythm. (I eventually got better at this, but it took a couple of years.) The painful consequence was accidents—a lot of them. Any day, at any time, I might look down and see a big wet spot between my legs or, worse yet, realize that I had involuntarily emptied my bowels. These accidents were so frequent that my mom had to be on call. I would track her down, wherever she was, and this was a time before pagers or cell phones. She would come get me, take me home, help me clean up, redress, and then take me back to school. There were some days when I couldn't find her right away, days when I would keep going to classes, pretending not to have the problem. Some of these days were as painful as any day I had in intensive care . . . just different.

I even had a bowel accident on the day that I gave a big speech in front of the whole school. I was running for student council president and wearing new, white pants and my dad's red V-neck sweater. It happened in the morning, and I had just enough time to make it home, clean up, put my clothes through the washer and dryer, make it back to school, and deliver my speech. The good news is that I made it in time and won the election. I was elected student council president at the end of eighth grade for the following year.

The painful side of returning to school was one that I kept away from my friends. They just saw the red sweater, white pants, and my smiling face.

The thud of the rock that nearly breaks me comes on November 16, just over two months into eighth grade. After nearly a year, I finally finished outpatient physical therapy yesterday. I am still hit-or-miss on transferring up from the floor, but I have mastered wheelies and going up small curbs and bumping my butt up a few stairs while sitting out of my wheelchair. Now, on Tuesdays and Thursdays, I can go home after school, just like any other kid.

It is Friday. Another week of school has ended and the excitement of the forthcoming weekend is knocking at the door. My brother and I are hanging out together. Since the addition to the house was completed, we are sharing a bedroom again. We are beginning to feel like fun-loving brothers again.

I am between our twin beds, my chair facing the headboards. While passing by, James begins to tickle me from behind under my arms. I am leaning forward, my torso pressing against the top of my thighs. I am giggling uncontrollably. Something happens, a spasm, something. My chair tips forward, and I am on my way down. I tuck my chin—what I was taught to do, but only if I was falling backward. As I tumble forward, my head hits awkwardly against the floor. I am lying on my side and stomach, my cheek pressing against the tan carpet. My arms are somehow caught underneath me; I can see only my right hand. I try to sit up by pushing my arms against the floor. Nothing. I look at my hand. It is twitching, opening and closing slightly. It is not my hand. It has become an object.

"James, call a doctor," my carpet-muffled voice squeaks out.

"What?"

"Call a doctor," I moan.

"Quit kidding around. It's not funny."

"James, I can't move my arms . . . something terrible has happened . . . I can't feel anything." My vision dims; sounds grow faint; my eyes close. Time is changing shape.

"You better not be kidding."

"James . . ." I break into sobs.

"Holy shit, holy shit. What should I do?" He is not asking; he is taking charge. He is being my older brother. He looks down at me folded on myself. Still in disbelief, he says, "Matt, I am going to pick you up . . . ready?" At this moment, I am paralyzed from the neck down; there is no way to object.

"James, be careful . . . it's my neck." He lifts my head and places it in the crook of his arm and begins to lift. Colors blur out the corners of my eyes. I am falling, dropping. There is nothing, no floor, no bottom, no base, a disorienting gap between my head and my body. I know this drop down a canyon; the last time, it was accompanied by plaster and metal racks and body casts. For an instant, I am dying once again. "My neck . . ." He lays me gingerly on the bed. I feel a load of bricks hitting concrete. "The pillow, move the pillow," I squeal. He sets my unfelt arms across my chest and rushes to the phone in the kitchen. Somehow, he tracks down Dr. Van Pufflen. An ambulance is called. We will meet him in the emergency room.

As I lie there, waiting for the ambulance, I feel crooked, not on the outside but on the inside. The ceiling looks so clean; my eyes feel so light. Something is twisted or bent or wedged on the right side of my neck. I can feel the pressure. I am barely maintaining against a tidal rush of fear. I can see my brother at the very left edge of my field of vision. James is sitting on the bed, feet on the floor. His elbows are pressed into his thighs, his forehead into his hands. He is staring downward. He is lost.

As time stretches into silence, we wait for the siren. In a moment of calm and dread, sensation resurfaces—burning pinpricks throughout my upper body, even my fingers. "James, I can feel stuff again." I wonder if he knows this is a good sign.

As I am loaded into the ambulance, I hear my mom's voice. She has just returned home from a long lunch. I cannot see her because my gaze is locked straight up into the blue sky again. I am braced and taped and fastened and flattened onto a wooden board. My head is moving nowhere. I can feel my mom and brother enveloped by silence. Once again, they stand and watch as people frantically work over my body. We are headed down another tunnel.

I wait alone in the emergency room. The doctors want to eliminate any temptation to turn my head, even if it is to connect eyes with a loved one. I am waiting for the consulting neurologist to weigh in on my case. Dr. Freeman is the father of a friend whom I played both baseball and basketball with. Now, the direction of my life will hinge on his diagnosis. Dr. Van Pufflen has already confirmed that I did, in fact, break my neck. The fracture is at the bottom, between the sixth and seventh cervical vertebrae. He does not want to speculate whether the damage will be permanent, hence Dr. Freeman's involvement. That my upper body feels like it is on fire is a good sign. Beyond that, he says little. These couple of hours spent waiting are the longest of my life.

I keep trying to move my arms. It's like having a fat lip: *Is it really swollen? I'd better check; it might be different this time.* I keep trying to move, keep telling myself that this can't be. Two spinal cord injuries in less than a year—what are the odds? Nobody's luck is this bad. I wait, terrified, and temporarily ward off my fear with incredulity. Suddenly, one of my arms responds, not much, but enough to notice. This is not miraculous; this is the world snapping back into the realm of the conceivable. I have tears, silent ones, because I am grateful that my life has some sense of proportion. There is only so much I can take.

The movement in my arms is increasing, but it is still partial. I can just barely move them; their new weight exceeds anything I have encountered. Only threads of muscle fibers are engaging against gravity, against bone, a shrill shrieking at best. The cost is excruciating, molten beads fired haphazardly to their destination. But at least the pain proves my ownership. By the time Dr. Freeman enters my picture, I am gaining confidence. Complete and utter disaster has been averted.

"Matt, you must have a star by your name," Dr. Freeman chirps in amazement. He is in the forefront; Dr. Van Pufflen waits behind, and my family is beyond him. "I'm not quite sure how, but the fracture at C7 did not severely impact your spinal cord. It's hard to see why, but, in my opinion, the damage you have sustained should not be permanent. Over time, there should be a full recovery." I can feel the relief wash through my mother and brother. They too have learned to trust nothing.

"How did this happen? I barely fell," I ask. Dr. Van Pufflen steps forward on cue.

"We think the rods in your back are the culprits. The fracture is just beyond the top of the rods, the first unsupported point. We think when you fell, the impact had nowhere to go. Anyone else's neck would have given some, simply flexed. Yours couldn't. So the full force of impact was delivered to the point of fracture."

"What's to stop this from happening again?" my mom interjects.

"Quite frankly, not falling like that again." This is not what I want to hear. It's bad enough that I have horrible balance, that a stiff breeze feels like enough to spill me out of my chair. Now I am fragile in a way that was beyond my imagination a few hours ago. The ground never looked so scary. I am one awkward fall from quadriplegia. How does one absorb such a feeling? Already, I am recoiling from my body, letting a new reality set in. My body can break from being tickled. What else do I need to know? "But remember," Dr. Freeman adds, "you've dodged a bullet. You're a lucky young man."

Relatively lucky.

∽

Ten days later I am still in the hospital, but some movement has returned. I can push a wheelchair for short distances. It is not my wheelchair, because my unresponsive fingers cannot grab the rims. Instead, I am using a hospital loaner again. Rubber knobs stick out from the rims and allow the heel of my hands to push. I have lost virtually all of my strength—just holding my arms up is a strain. The more time my recovery takes, the more strength will be lost. I will be starting over. Physical therapy will begin again and weight lifting will begin again, all accompanied by burning pinpricks. When will this be over? I am ready to cash it in.

Right before Thanksgiving, I turn to my mom and try to make a joke.

"I guess it looks like we'll spend another Christmas in the hospital. Two in a row," I say, my head shaking with a faint, deadened smile. She knows what this means, that I am ready to give up. More than that, she knows that I am ready not to care.

A mother, when saving her child, is fierce, focused, and ready for action. She walks out of the room and calls a meeting with the staff. Her message is clear. "Start telling Matt he will be going home soon, that he will not be staying in the hospital much longer." My mother is picking up the pieces once again, but this time not aimlessly, like at the scene of the car accident. Now, she is determined not to lose either of her sons.

My brother is also struggling. He lives with an incredible juxtaposition. He walks and I wheel. And now, he has been party to a horrific event, one that threatens to dissolve his younger brother. There is no blame, there is only what happened. He did not break my neck—it broke; the rods broke it. But his loving heart is shadowed by a potentially consuming guilt. He needs me to be all right. My mother is fighting for both of her sons.

Within a week, I am home. In another week, I am laboring to push myself down the halls at school, able to hold a pencil and even return to my typing class. (I was given a "mercy" B, with extenuating circumstances being cited.) I will fully recover over a period of five months. Physical therapy continues through the winter and into the first hints of spring. The main impact of this injury is not physical, however. I am pushed farther out of my body. Within my flesh, I carry metal objects that threaten me at every curb, during any loss of balance, during any collision with the floor. Being playful with my body is out, so is tickling, so is the relationship I know best with my brother. I move forward into my relatively lucky life with a deep mistrust of my body and an inward presence that continues to diminish.

11

Above the Chest

When Dr. Goff told me—in that final consultation when I first left the hospital—that if I was diligent, I could expect a relatively normal life, I felt a little more dead. And yet a relatively normal life is exactly what I set out to prove that I had. The years between ages fourteen and twenty-five, between breaking my neck and beginning yoga, were an attempt to live a normal life despite the traumatic rupture I experienced between my mind and body. For a long time, I generally succeeded.

As mentioned, I returned to school and became a leader in my class. I reestablished myself as a virtually straight-A student. In senior high school, I was treasurer of the Student Forum not once, but twice. Upon graduation, I won a local topflight scholarship to the college of my choice, one that paid me $3,600 a year for four years. I wore crewneck sweaters and boat shoes, and worked to succeed in the eyes of those around me. I imagined—along with everyone else—that I would become an attorney like my father, maybe even run for public office. On the outside, I strove to become the all-American product of my predominately white, Midwestern community.

I also had a steady stream of girlfriends. Looking back now, it was probably too steady. I was decent-looking enough, but the wheelchair, the disability—I was afraid it might keep me from experiencing intimacy with a woman. I went out of my way to prove otherwise. I sought to make my connections with girls more mature, more meaningful. I listened, I cared, I shared, and I laughed more deeply than most teenagers. I was selective, intuitively looking for depth, along with good looks, in potential girlfriends. When all was said and done, I pursued only one girl who was not ready to date a guy in a wheelchair. The downside of my approach was that I landed myself in some relatively serious relationships for a kid my age. Consequently, I think I missed some of the fun of high school.

I also became sexually active during this time—it was the last great uncertainty of paraplegia, or at least it seemed so to me. I can't say it was great sex, but few can as a teenager. It was a bit clumsy and took a lot of communication with my partner about how things were different for me. It's hard for anyone to talk about sex, let alone kids at that age. But this forced communication also put my sexuality on novel footing. Sex for me was not a lusty, backseat experience. It had to be planned, thought about, and discussed. Even in these first few experiences, I was beginning to learn something that I have carried with me for a lifetime. Sexual expression is a shared exploration of intimacy and bodies. One consequence of my spinal cord injury has been a de-emphasizing of the central role played by sexual intercourse. While I am capable of it and even enjoy it, there is so much more to sexual intimacy than an explosion of physical sensation between the legs. I doubt that I would have known this as deeply had I not been a paraplegic.

〜

After spending my first year of college in Duluth, I chose to follow in my parents' and my brother's footsteps to the University of Minnesota in the Twin Cities. Never mind that the winters in Minnesota have always been brutal, that the U of M has one of the biggest campuses in the country, and that getting from class to class would take extraordinary effort. These considerations did not matter. I unconsciously wanted to prove my relatively normal life. My measuring stick—the life I would have had.

Something didn't feel right, though. While the promise of a relatively normal life did not particularly inspire me, the issue went deeper than that. My life thus far had been anything but normal. Something had happened to me—not just the accident, not just the loss of my father and sister or my ensuing paralysis—something else had happened too. I felt like I had been left with a secret, an insight about living and dying. I could not articulate what it was, but I did have a nagging sense of what it was not.

It was not to simply live a relatively normal life. I felt far too weighty, too heavy, like there was a purpose to what I had experienced. My inward silence had also driven a wedge between my "relatively normal" achievements and my sense of accomplishment, not unlike when I stopped playing video games in the hospital. I felt hollow in what I was doing, not prideful or joyous. It would take years for me to realize that the silence itself was the insight I was sensing, that it held the key to what I was seeking.

In the meantime, I felt compelled to move my life in a different direction. In retrospect, I know now that the silence I carried within me was also coming unglued. Over the next five years or so, my perception became increasingly negative. I became disillusioned with the world, our country, our choices. Eventually, this negativity made it impossible for me not to seek a different path—after all, I was born with a smile on my face. Paradoxically, this difficult period also marked the beginning of my efforts to heal the dislocation between my mind and my body.

My twentieth year proved to be an important one. The change of direction in my life began with a powerful dream. I was a sophomore at the U of M. I lived with four other guys and was having a ball. Although we took studying seriously, we also didn't miss any opportunity to be young and stupid. It was winter quarter. I was generally exhausted from trudging day after day around a snow-laden campus.

During a much-needed afternoon nap, I had this startling dream. I am sitting at my family's dining room table. I am on one side and a whole slew of people are on the other. My sister is sitting directly across from me; everyone else is standing. I feel the heart-lifting warmth of a family get-together. Laura and I are chatting underneath the party banter. I can feel the smooth depth of her intonation, as if she is whispering in my ear. I feel deeply contented. Suddenly, I notice that the people standing behind her are my relatives. But more than that, they are my dead relatives—both of my grandfathers, my maternal grandmother, and others I can feel but do not know. They are all smiling at me. Once I realize that they are dead, their faces begin to dissolve, their bodies transform into a transparent presence. Laura maintains her form the longest. She floats across the table and gives me a wonderful hug. I can feel her—her smell, her loving kindness against my chest. As she releases me, I feel her whisper, "I'll see you in four years." I am so thankful. I have missed her terribly.

I wake up feeling that I have received a precious gift. I can literally feel the imprint of my sister against my chest. Who knows what ghosts are? Who knows what dreams are? I had just touched my sister in what felt like three dimensions. I am not doubting what happened; the experience is mine. But then, out of nowhere, I am enveloped by fear. *Wait a minute, what did she mean by four years?* Possibly she meant that she would return, that we would touch again. But what if she meant I would be joining her, joining my dead relatives? I become still. This late afternoon suddenly feels different, the things in my room—my desk, my discarded clothes, my wheelchair parked next to my bed—become a muted kind of new. Feeling the possibility of my own death, I feel survival take hold.

After much pining, I decide on an interpretation, a healing story. Laura would never burden me with the awareness of my own death. But she would warn me of an impending choice. I end up deciding that both of my initial reactions are potentially true. In four years, she will either take me with her or we will share another visit. I feel my survival is on the line and I need to choose—am I to move toward living or let myself continue to dwindle away? At twenty, I did not know how to react to such a thing, how to imagine that a dream can provide a pivotal message. But I knew that I had to do something.

At the end of this winter quarter, I switched my major from history—a clear-cut path toward law school—to philosophy. This signified more than a change of subjects. It was evidence of my growing belief that I had an insight to share, something that mattered. I thought I could explore what I was feeling through the study of philosophy.

Switching majors was also an acknowledgment that I didn't have enough answers, that I needed to start asking more questions. This went directly against the underpinnings of my male, relatively normal life. Up until that point, I knew that I had much to learn, but I still possessed an underlying confidence that I knew how the world worked and what it needed. By opening myself to a wider spectrum of thoughts, to even questioning the basic components of reality, I upended that confidence and altered the course of my life.

My interest in philosophy, both in undergraduate and graduate studies, focused on the mind-body problem and issues related to consciousness. Without knowing it, I was beginning the process of reconnecting to my body. But at this point, I still believed what the doctors had told me at age thirteen—that there was no way to reconnect to my paralyzed body short of a regenerated spinal cord. This meant that to access my paralyzed body in a more living, engaged way, I needed a paradigm shift. I had to literally change my relationship to the world. Without knowing exactly what I was doing and why, I took a shot-gun approach—I began to question almost everything I had ever been told in my entire life.

At the same time, however, the switch to philosophy went against the practical vigor of my upbringing. Earning a living and providing for a family is a mainstay of a relatively normal life. And quite frankly, a lifelong pursuit of philosophy did not bode well for reasonable income generation.

Luckily, this tension was lessened for me. A few years earlier, my family had brought a lawsuit against the state of Iowa for negligence concerning our accident. We successfully argued that the Department of Transportation had violated their own guidelines when building the slope of the embankment down which our car tumbled. They also had violated their own guidelines concerning when to sand Interstate 35, the road on which our family was driving. This second issue came down to an ill-advised decision by a sand-truck driver not to sand on the morning of November 26, 1978. He hit his snooze button and rolled over—beginning the innocent unfolding of an accident. The result was that not one, but three cars slid down that embankment within a span of twenty minutes. Our family sustained the only serious injuries.

How my mom came to bring the lawsuit is a story in itself. My recollection is that one day, less than two years after the accident, I asked a simple question around our dinner table: "Why weren't there guard rails?" We mused about this for a while, shrugged our shoulders, and went back to using our forks. A short time later, my mom had a dream or a vision or something. In it, she was speaking with my father. He told her to initiate a lawsuit and told her to hurry. Keyed into the "openness" left by trauma, she obliged and called my father's law firm. With a last-minute scramble, we filed on the final day before the two-year statute of limitations ran out.

By seventeen years of age, I was awarded, through a settlement, a hefty sum of money. It was for the damage done to my body, to my life's arc. My mother was compensated for the loss of her breadwinner husband, and she also received a minimal amount for the death of my sister. Apparently, because Laura was only twenty and did not have an established profession, there was no basis upon which to assess her value. My brother was not a claimant in the suit. Legally, the courts do not recognize damages that cannot be measured, ones that travel strictly on the inside. He was again asked to stand on his own.

At the time, the money changed virtually nothing for me. I was firmly planted on my path of a relatively normal life. I invested the money, spending only what I needed to spend, for example, paying for costs associated with college. I kept the rest in a rainy-day fund—what if I need a drastic medical procedure, what if there is a miracle cure for spinal cord injuries? The money went into a mental compartment labeled "in case of the unthinkable."

At twenty, I began to think differently, though. It dawned on me that there was enough money that, if I maintained a modest standard of living, I could live off of my investments. This afforded me the luxury of asking a basic, life-guiding question: How can I give back to the world? My initial answer was to start thinking—through the study of philosophy—about a world that felt increasingly out of joint, a world that was missing something essential. Of course, what was really missing was my body, but worrying about the world was safer.

⁊

About a year later, as a junior in college, I have what is—for lack of a better word—an episode. It is winter again. I am driving to get my girlfriend; she will be spending the night at my place. This eerie Sunday night has almost no traffic. A week-old snowfall is now greasy and dirty. I am driving above the ice-laden Mississippi River on the Franklin Avenue Bridge. This bridge feels tired. Once a vibrant spoke of bustle and traffic in an emerging economy, now it is an overlooked passageway, a relic pushed aside by sprawling metropolitan freeways. The three-block drive feels like traveling through time.

I am wondering if Jane and I will have sex tonight. The image I carry of myself regarding who I am supposed to be—a fun-loving, hormone-driven college student—is in conflict with reality. In truth, I am not led by my loins. For me, for sex to be truly enjoyable, it requires enhanced focus, the conscious appreciation of the subtleties of lovemaking—all the things that actually matter. It cannot be brainless. It must be serious, and serious is not what I want just now. I start thinking about my body, about how mine is so different. I feel the contrast between my loins and walking loins—my loss of movement . . . loss. My dread begins as tragic appreciation. *How strange my life is,* I say to myself. Soon I am imagining that the presence I experience within my body is on display, lit up by lights. I imagine an uninjured body next to mine; it is also lighted. In comparison, so much of me has become dark. I feel a creeping loss of light, of growing older. But mine is accelerated; from the nipple line down, I am already gone, two-thirds of me is already snuffed out. This perceived acceleration of losing space, of losing ground, consumes me. I am only twenty-one. As I am driving, I am breathing less, becoming less. Inwardly, I moan, *Why am I being pushed out of life?* Seized with dread, I pull over on this forgotten bridge, press my head against the steering wheel, and cry without tears.

I am without tears because I am reaching for my most familiar healing story: using the silence to achieve a deadened acceptance. I am not pounding the steering wheel; that would be angry. I am not sobbing; that would be realized grief. Instead, I close my eyes, feel my head upon the wheel, feel a sudden quiet within my car. I mutter, *This is my life . . . this is what it is.* Of course, I am not breathing when I think these words. I am static, gripped in the space after exhalation, giving a life-denying offering to the life that is mine. Once the silence deadens me, I can reboot with the tragic feeling of a broken life and a decision to willfully live anyway.

This moment is more than eight years in the making, a culmination of negative healing stories, beginning with the doctor's prescribed unreality of phantom feelings. As I continue my drive along this particular bridge, on this particular night, I have completely become an upper torso—the rest of my body is dead. I am no longer trying to make the rehabilitation's healing vision work. I am it. My head, neck, arms, and chest sleep with Jane that night. We do not have sex, and the relationship begins to end.

So when does healing begin? Perhaps this negative realization of losing "space" within my body pushes me over a threshold. Life as an upper torso is unacceptable; my survival begins to rouse itself once again. This does not mean there are immediate results. I do not go *ding* like a perky microwave oven and suddenly reconfigure within my body. Still more pressure is required.

Over time, a phase begins where I manifest gray. I wear almost exclusively gray clothes; I buy a gray car with a gray interior. I live in a gray, north-facing apartment, tucked into a gigantic, characterless complex. I have the interior of my next living space—one side of a duplex bought with my brother—painted gray. I buy gray carpet. I unconsciously create a world that mirrors how I inwardly feel. My smile even deadens for what will be years. I become negatively aware of the world around me, of the values that I was reared with, of the folly of human beings. I apply to graduate schools, a stressful process in itself. I notice that my hands hurt, both of them in the same place, the space between the knuckles of my pinky and ring fingers. One day, I realize that the pain is self-inflicted. I have been unconsciously rolling my own knuckles, wringing my hands as I ruminate on the plight of living. But it is my living that is being denied, not the world's.

Of course, the hardest times also begin healing. Living and dying occur simultaneously. During this gray period, I find my first and most important bodyworker and begin the search for my lost body. Carole is in her late thirties and has red henna highlights in her hair. She wears purple, drinks tea, and is perhaps the most intuitive person I have ever met.

A bodyworker lies outside of my paradigm, but I need something, something to shake me loose. Carole does massage, but that is not her specialty. She practices a blend of various methods, but her focus is on influencing the flow of energy through the body. She introduces me to many new concepts: energy body, trigger points, muscle testing, chakras, tuning forks, and others. But she does not teach me in two dimensions—through talking and words. Instead, she shows me—through my body—how to release the physical and mental trauma that I hold. Of course, the trained philosopher in me is skeptical, but over time, he too must sit back and observe the awareness that begins to unfold through my body.

With Carole's help, I begin to acknowledge the price my body has paid. It has taken more than ten years, but I am ready to acknowledge just how damaged I am, how difficult my life is. My will is tired, my body is tired, and my mind finally admits to living in a protracted survival mode. It is not a relatively normal life. I am beginning to surrender.

Most important, Carole shows me that my paralyzed body has not fallen silent. It did not die. Rather, it changed its voice, speaking now on a subtler frequency but still offering keys to its inner experience. Carole radically affects how I view my body and bodies generally. She sets the groundwork, the framework, for my future yoga practice. She teaches me to listen inwardly to energy, to its movement. She gives me my first access to my whole body again. I am forever grateful.

I also fall in love during this gray time, knockdown, flat-out in love. Somebody sees me, not my relatively normal shell, but me. It is Liz, my first wife. She whispers to me that I am an angel, that I am trying to land. Although she shares my pessimistic view of the world and adds a feminist perspective, she helps me feel subtlety and magic and the ageless wisdom of women. She listens to great music, loves eating chocolate, and wears high-top Converse sneakers. She brings both a playful and a serious depth to my life.

On September 30, 1989, when I am not quite twenty-four, Liz and I marry. After our wedding in the Twin Cities, we immediately move to Santa Barbara. We begin our married life, away from our friends, in a new city and in the midst of my beginning graduate school in philosophy at the University of California at Santa Barbara. Our four years of marriage is another story, as is our divorce—ones that I will not be telling. Just know that I was in love and that we are still friends.

⌐

Two events—one big, one small—are the straws that push me toward the healing of yoga. The first occurs during my second year of graduate school. It is January 1991. I am twenty-five. Our country cunningly executes the ground-war portion of the Persian Gulf War—Operation Desert Storm—in four days. Through the media, our leaders brag about there being only 140-plus casualties. But in the vacant vision behind my eyes, I see piles and piles of more than 100,000 Iraqi people dead. I hear the silence of their abandoned bodies, real people lost, real families changed forever. As the media follows General H. Norman Schwarzkopf's celebrity tour, I feel like I am living in a cartoon. The bite of the absurdity fuels an overwhelming sense of death.

Simultaneously, I am taking a graduate seminar in epistemology— the philosophical study of human knowledge. We are reading Plato's *Theaetetus,* the famous dialogue in which Socrates puts forward the notion that knowledge is true justified belief. Basically, this means that a belief counts as knowledge if it is true and if we can provide good, sound reasons for believing it. We talk about this for ten straight weeks. We piss and piddle, and labor and argue. We indulge in the exercise of abstract thinking and, worse yet, make ourselves believe it matters. Bombs are dropping, lives are ripping, talking heads are boasting, and here I am. The juxtaposition makes me nauseous.

After winter quarter, I take a leave of absence from school. I tell my graduate advisor, "I have to take care of my body. I'm coming apart." Of course, it is my mind that is coming apart, because most of my body has already been abandoned.

The other event happens shortly thereafter. A stray cat starts hanging around my house. He is dangerously skinny, with bald spots plopped throughout his already sparse fur. At first, this cat is an annoyance, sleeping on my front stoop, holding me hostage with his needful meows. Over the course of days, he moves to the backyard and the back stairs. I grow accustomed to his company. I make him a soft bed in a low-sided box, buy cat food, and coax him back to the dignity of the front stoop. He will not eat or drink water. I realize that he is preparing to die, and I am not ready. I rush him to the vet, but there is nothing to do. His kidneys have shut down, and he has no teeth. He is suffering. Suddenly, I am confronted by a different story, one that is out of my control. This worn-out old cat is sharing his death, choosing me as his witness. I make another vet appointment; I will help him sleep. As my hand rests gently on his side, we wait for the injection. He is quiet, his breathing shallow. Maybe I just met this cat; maybe we are old friends; maybe it doesn't matter. I wonder as the flicker leaves his eyes. I am stricken with unrealized grief. It is time for yoga.

Part Three
Yoga, Bodies, and Baby Boys

12

Taking My Legs Wide

I met my yoga teacher, Jo Zukovich, on the third Saturday of April in 1991, more than twelve years after the accident. I was still on a leave of absence from my graduate studies. She was teaching a weekend workshop at the Aikido Center. A woman I knew got us connected. Maia was a body-worker, a brown belt in aikido, and about to begin studying as a midwife. One day, as she gave me a massage, she casually asked if I would be interested in trying yoga. She set up a meeting with Jo, who taught in San Diego but made the trek to Santa Barbara once every six weeks.

As I approached the aikido dojo that day, it was sunny and unusually bright. I had no idea what to expect, no idea if yoga was even possible for a paralyzed person. When I rolled up to the doorway, I heard no voices, nothing. Was I at the right place? Was this where I was supposed to be? I didn't dare look in. To make my apprehension worse, there was a tattoo shop above the dojo, and out of its windows was blaring Pink Floyd's *Dark Side of the Moon*. A more surreal frame for this experience would be hard to imagine. This was the moment before my life would make an unexpected turn, a moment with sun, music, and me hovering uneasily at the door.

⌇

Did my path to yoga begin that day? Life's experiences are all open to interpretation, stories willing to be told. I have already hinted at other possible entry points into yoga. My overt out-of-body experience began something; those four twisting screws created a beginning glimpse into a separating silence between mind and body, a silence that now underpins my experience with yoga. Did something start when I began using the silence within my paralyzed body as a protective barrier against pain? Perhaps it really began when a thirteen-year-old boy was guided to forsake his paralyzed body. At the early dawn of maturity, life threw me off-track and gave me a lifetime dislocation between mind and body. Did this begin the opposite of yoga and thus lead me inevitably to it? When does a path begin?

I am young, no more than five. The year is 1970. My father has been in a series of minor car accidents. I am told that he has sustained something called whiplash and is in a lot of pain. Nothing seems to help. Eventually, he begins to practice this weird kind of exercising. Early in the morning, he sets a plastic mat over the gold plush carpet in my parents' bedroom. It reminds me of the game Twister. He sits in his boxer shorts, centered on the mat, and quietly pages through a book filled with pictures. After some study, he strains and grunts his inflexible body into odd shapes and positions. It doesn't look like fun, and yet I am fascinated by the quiet intensity of his focus. Day after day, I watch his regimen: the rhythm of his breath, the glistening of sweat, the sound of skin rubbing against plastic mat. Not allowed to speak, my experience grows in mystery. Each day, he wipes off with a towel, neatly folds up his mat, and places it—along with the book—into the front left corner of his closet. Then off to a shower, a shave, and a day's work.

For me, the wonder of what he does resides in that book. The cover is yellow, with a picture of a dark-skinned man sitting in a strange position. It is not long before I start sneaking into his closet to steal peeks at those alluring pages. I am both attracted and horrified. In one picture, the man's whole body is parallel to the floor as he balances only on his hands. It looks like magic. But there are other pictures. The man is kneeling on the soles of his feet, palms turned upward, hands spread widely over his knees. His eyes are bulging out of their sockets, and his tongue is sticking down past the bottom of his chin. He looks insane. As I am prone to nightmares, I quickly turn the pages. But then comes the unimaginable. The man is sitting in simple cross-legs, and each hand is holding the end of a thick string—it looks more like a round shoelace. The string—to my horror—goes into his nose and out his mouth. Not surprisingly, his eyes are again bulging. It gives me chills. Still, I find myself looking at this book quite often, both to touch what my dad is practicing and for a good spooking in the middle of my childhood day.

Thirty-three years later, I have that very book in front of me.

My mom came across it a couple of years ago. She thinks she bought it for my dad at a rummage sale. Knowing what I know now, I realize that the book was intended to sensationalize yoga, to shock the Western reader or any five-year-old voyeur sitting in his dad's closet. Published in 1957, this book was part of an initial wave of yogic awareness in the West. It did nothing to change the image of yoga as an esoteric art composed of strange and bizarre practices. In fact, it banked on it.

As I hold this book and travel through my memories, I am amazed by what my father was doing: his willingness to explore, the discipline needed to learn from a book, his solitary attempt to transform his life. They all stir me deeply. Still walking off his family farm, he pursued yoga long before it was in fashion, long before its commonsense approach to possessing a mind and a body had filtered into our popular culture. Knowing what I know now, I want to support him on his path, to help him with his poses, to let him ask the questions I know he had. The serious study of yoga requires a teacher. I cannot even imagine not having met Jo, not having her gentle guidance or sharp words at just the right times.

That man, sitting on his plastic mat in 1970, was lonely. His search had brought him to a place he didn't quite grasp, one that lacked the reassurance of a clearly traveled path in front of him. I have my own version of that loneliness. I, too, am searching for something transformative. While I do have a yoga teacher, we have never lived in the same city. While I do practice where yoga is more widely accepted, I do so from within a paralyzed body. I do not know where the work is going, or even what is possible. But, while the work may be solitary, the impetus comes from loving the world, from wanting to join it. I wonder if he knew this, too.

I wait nervously on the sidewalk outside the dojo to meet my yoga teacher for the first time. Like after every yoga class, people are lingering, not with anything in particular to say, but with a shapeless need. Something has been shared, an insight, an uncommon intimacy. If the dispersion is too quick, the shared connection feels lost and the world becomes smaller once again. My entrance into the dojo adds confusion and curiosity. Confusion because there is a step and someone who has never bumped a wheelchair up a step must now do so. Curiosity because that same wheelchair, along with the person in it, is coming to meet the teacher.

Within this cloud of awkward transition, Jo and I meet each other's gaze. A silence is shared, a relief. The feeling that it's going to be fine moves through our bodies. This is felt before words, before details. I am already her student.

Inside the door, there is a three-foot entryway and a bench for sitting. Then another step up. The rest of the dojo's floor is covered with a hard white mat. No shoes, let alone wheels, traverse this ground. This is a place where bodies tumble and twist and fall. A martial art is practiced here, and its imprint is tangibly felt.

But now there is another problem. "Can you get down on the mat?" Jo asks.

I pause with uncertainty. I didn't expect to be separated from my wheelchair so quickly. "I can get down, but who knows about up."

She nods and smiles. "Obviously, there is plenty of help around."

Jo is in her mid-forties, but her body is years younger. She wears a toe ring, funky bracelets, and shoulder-length strawberry blonde hair. Powerfully connected with the ground, her strength is wound tightly, like a pit bull's sturdy stance. And yet, she is graceful and supple and thinks nothing of pointing with her feet. More than anything, her body is her own. Already I am learning. During our private session, she sits on the floor with me, catches my gaze, and asks me to sit as straight as possible. I smile and confidently tell her that I am. In truth, my body is so very injured, so out of alignment. My right foot is nearly three inches in front of my left. My weight sits unevenly on my right hip, and my upper body hunches to the left in compensation. My shoulders are far from level. But in my mind's eye, this is straight.

Jo has never worked with someone with a spinal cord injury. Intuitively, she knows to move slowly, gently, to not make me confront my lost body too quickly. "Can you put your hands slightly behind you and lift your chest? Good. Now can you do it again, but this time don't hold your breath?" I'm a little alarmed— *How does she know?* Oh well, the work continues.

"Can you take your legs wide, like a big V?" she says. The spasticity in my legs resists, but eventually they spread and stay put. I am hit by a rush of something, something feels strange, something . . . "Matt, can you put your hands on your thighs, lift your chest, and breathe?" The rush intensifies. I feel something, like I am floating—no, flying. Suddenly, it hits me. This is the first time in over twelve years that my legs have been wide. The strange feeling I am experiencing is the rush of lost time. My eyes close, my voice choking, "My legs haven't been this wide since . . ." Jo bows her head and whispers, "I know."

What we have shared cannot be undone. She has seen, more clearly than anyone has, into what I have lost. Her strength holds firm. We have love at first purpose. She is my teacher; I am her student. We will work through a lifetime. She knows to keep moving. "Matt, can you put your hands in prayer? Keep your elbows at your sides. Stretch from your shoulders to your elbows, from your elbows to your wrists. Press your palms together, stretch through each finger, and lift your chest." I am struck again. The pose seals itself, completes a sense of energetic connection. My chest seems to lift effortlessly, a feeling of lightness releases out the top of my head. Jo sees what I am experiencing. "That's amazing, especially for your first time," she says. Now we both know that I will be a good student.

That I could feel such things so quickly—the loud rush produced by simply taking my legs wide, the upward energetic release produced when hands-in-prayer was done with yogic precision— meant that those phantom feelings had not left me. Instead, they had been waiting in the silence, waiting for me to let them back into my conscious experience. Consciousness does not abandon us. It is only denied.

My life seems to have prepared me for my first encounter with Jo, again like a river gaining current. Before meeting her, I had been surviving on slim rations when it came to body experience. I was ready for a prison break.

When yogic instruction rekindled a feeling of energetic sensation within my mind-body relationship, it felt like settling into a warm bath—the relief, the feeling of nourishment, the calm and quieting reference. I grew in dimension as my *entire* body began whispering to me once again, albeit in a more eloquent voice.

The splendor and subtlety of living is most apparent in the conscious presence of the silence. Now, after thirteen years of yoga practice, not only do I feel an upward energetic release in hands-in-prayer, I also feel a downward energetic connection to the earth. Is this the same as being able to perform a complex, pretzel-shaped physical pose? Obviously not. Progress is what you make of it.

After this first encounter, Jo sends me home with these simple poses, plus one more. "Shaking hands with your feet" is not a pose exactly. It is an act, a ritual, an introduction. I am to take my foot, put a finger between each of my toes, and form a clasp. Then I am to rock and gently roll the ball of my foot first in one direction and then another. I am to "shake hands" with my feet. Sounds simple, right? This will become one of the hardest poses for me to do. The hurdle is not physical. I have been consciously ignoring my lower body for more than twelve years.

There is a gulf of silence a mile wide between my feet and me. They feel like a foreign country. I pretend that shaking hands with my feet is no big deal, just a movement like putting one foot in front of the other. Underneath, though, the river is different, the symbolic healing is so acute, so direct that I feel nauseous, like getting out of bed too fast. I do not consciously avoid this pose. Instead, it strikes me as stupid, a silly waste of time. "I want to do the real stuff," I tell myself. This pose will not become a habit for years.

Before I can begin the "real" stuff, I have problems to solve. First, there are wood floors in my house. After twelve years of paralysis, I have a bony butt—the dissolving atrophy of inaction. The sound of my sits bones (the bones in my butt) rolling unprotected over a hard surface is like fingernails scratching down a blackboard, unnatural enough to cause a three-dimensional shiver. I go to a sporting goods store and buy two one-inch-thick, six-foot-long, deep blue exercise mats. On them is a picture of a perky woman wearing workout tights, a headband, and an affected smile. She glistens happily with sweat and looks like she might break into a dance-line high step at any moment. *Life must be good in that body,* I mentally mumble, but I do not believe her. *What does she know—she has no idea.* My resisting mind searches for ways to make what I am doing feel wrong. Maybe I should be embarrassed to buy what is advertised as a woman's exercise mat. I'm a guy, and home-centered self-improvement offends my socialized sense of manliness. Still, I buy the protection for my butt and awkwardly tote the mats to my car.

The real problem is how I am going to move between the floor and my wheelchair. It is an incredibly difficult transfer. A dead lift of a paralyzed body requires brutish strength. There is no easy place from which to lift, no place to secure a leveraged and balanced point of exertion. My shoulders are not flexible enough for both of my hands to reach the level of my seat. If one hand stays on the floor while the other pushes from the seat, the lift lacks direction and my legs flop awkwardly off-center. This drives me to frustration rather than my butt into the chair. I do not possess Dwight-like strength to compensate for my shortcomings in balance and grace.

The thought of having to do this transfer on a daily basis makes my head spin. Enter the blue velvet chair. It sits innocently in the corner, its seat much lower than the seat height of my wheelchair. It is stained, the velvet's nap dried and pushed against its natural grain. This chair will become instrumental in my early relationship with yoga. In retrospect, I romantically imagine that this chair was waiting for me, waiting for me to realize its place: a step up and into a new world. It becomes a place for me to think and practice yoga through the difficult times that wait ahead.

For now, however, I am scratching my head, trying to figure out how I am going to get off the floor. That's when I truly see the blue velvet chair for the first time. Why must I make it back into my wheelchair in one fell swoop? How did I get stuck in this all-or-nothing loop? Such a simple thought is a revelation. I have nothing to prove, no increase in physical strength is necessary for me to move forward. Rather, I can think, problem solve, and find my own way back from the floor. My new mats fold in half. I can stack them on top of each other and easily hoist myself up to that height. From there, I can make it onto the blue velvet chair, pull my wheelchair around, and make the difficult transfer back to my mobility. It may not be pretty or powerful or inspiring, but it works.

Finding the floor and a way back is healing. It may sound too simple, too easy to lift a damaged heart. But most of our shackles are invisible. I am leaving my wheelchair via a blue velvet chair. This is healing.

Taking my legs wide and realizing the blue velvet chair were breakthroughs. Both were steps back toward the ordinary, back toward a life where common sense has traction. My body deserves to live in more spaces, not fewer. So what if my life as a paraplegic does not require that my legs go wide. Does that mean they never should? That would be like never watching a sunset because it has no practical function. Taking my legs wide was a return to common sense. So too was using the blue velvet chair. I was a paraplegic and there was a certain way (with speed and will) that I had been guided to do things. This vision ran deep, so much so that I had never contemplated using small steps to get back up into my chair. Performing this simple action began to release me from the grip of a limiting healing vision. Suddenly, my body began to present other possibilities—the beginning of yogic realization.

13

Body Memories

I have a mishap while doing yoga on my own for only the second time. Anticipation has gotten the best of me. It is early, and I want to get started. The chill of California spring finds easy passage through the uninsulated walls of my rented adobe house. The wood floor creaks with every shift of my weight. I feel like I am finally doing something, finally working to live through my entire body.

The pose I am doing is called *dandasana,* translated from the Sanskrit as "staff of life." The classic instructions are simple: Sit with your legs straight out in front of you, press your palms into the floor beside your hips, and lift your chest. Jo has modified it slightly so that my hands are a little farther behind me. I cannot hold the pose very long because lifting my chest subtly changes the directional exertion of my diaphragm. It is enough to rob my ignored body of its breath. Still, I push forward. As I lift my chin up toward the ceiling, making the energy of the pose approach that of a backbend, something slips and catches painfully at the base of my neck. My right arm is shot full of tingles. Fear pulses through me.

Gingerly, I sit up straight and start to flex my hand and arm. Thankfully, they still work. But I have lost the normal feeling in two of my fingers to the sensation of pinpricks. I am dangerously close to a much bigger problem. The only thing I can figure out is that the Harrington rods in my upper back have slipped and are now pinching a nerve. This turns out to be exactly the case.

Since causing my neck to break at age fourteen, I have learned to avoid these rods. My posture has become a miracle of passive contortion. My shoulders have rolled forward and scrunched toward my ears. My head has jutted out away from my torso; my chin has turned slightly upward. I have unconsciously created a protective dead zone at the base of my neck. In short, the rods and I have entered into a postural nonaggression pact. I stay out of the troubled area, and the rods will injure me no more than they already have. Truce.

Starting yoga broke this pact. I consult with an orthopedic surgeon. The pinched nerve at the base of my neck will clear up on its own. The rods, however, pose a different problem. They were originally inserted into my back for support while the bone fusion solidified. That process was complete in about two years. Now, the rods only pose a threat to increased activity in my neck and upper back. The only solution is surgical removal. The upshot is that to pursue yoga, I will have to purge metal.

The surgery is scheduled for the beginning of June, a little over a month away. Before performing the procedure, the surgeon insists that I embark on a month of physical therapy. He wants the muscles in my upper back to strengthen and loosen up before being traumatized again.

⌖

Why is yoga so important? Is it worth having major surgery? Even before I experience the practical benefits of yoga, the rods present powerful resistance. This waiting period gives me ample time to think. The rods feel symbolic. They are vestiges of the death that I absorbed so many years earlier. Their inanimate metal represents a lifeless past and stands between me and where I want to go. I want to scream, "Get this shit out of my body!" But I am also begging the rods to leave, pleading, because I am scared. They have cast such a powerful shadow over my life these last twelve years.

I also question what I hope to gain from the practice of yoga. How could it transform a paralyzed body, a body that can do only a limited number of poses? While in the midst of these doubts, I have an experience that helps me move forward.

I am lying flat on my back in my backyard. My arms are wide, my eyes are closed, and I am set upon moist, strawlike spring grass. As the California sun warms my face, I am letting part of me die. The toil, the will, the arms that dragged my body to this time, to this place, must sleep. Years and years of hollowing struggle are releasing into the ground. This is what I believe; this is what I am imagining.

I am being covered—the shovel's nose crisply cutting the earth, the sound of thrown soil encasing my body, the smell of open dirt. I am becoming buried so I can rest, so I can wake, so I can begin again. As the dirt covers my face, my dreamlike vision dims. I feel the earth's benevolent hum. I drift off to sleep.

When I awake, I decide to plant my first garden. My landlord has recently cut down an ailing orange tree; he has even ground out the stump. All that remains is a bald patch, six feet in diameter, waiting for me. I need a beginning, something tangible to help me feel the paradigm shift required to rebuild my life. I decide on a garden.

The ground needs tilling and I cannot work such a machine. I decide to use my hands, to feel the dirt directly. Soon my tilling takes a backseat to observation. Where I expect nothing but plain, lifeless dirt, I encounter just the opposite. The amount of living in this soil is staggering—gruesome acts of carnage, feats of incredible strength, even occasional cooperation. Most of all, there is a continuous bustle of life. Despite having their world literally turned inside out, the grubs, bugs, and insects don't miss a beat. They embody a singleness of purpose, a theme within inflicted chaos. So seamless and rhythmic is their effort that they seem an outer expression of the earth's inner breathing.

Eventually my hands come upon a pile of bones, someone's kitten or hamster, maybe. I sink with the sense of having entered a forbidden place. Unearthing a grave feels like sacrilege—an interruption of a secret between the earth and its fallen child. And yet, the earth makes no judgment. She absorbs the bones of death with the same graceful presence that she houses grubs, bugs, and insects. Life and death side-by-side, unfazed and unassuming in a perpetual stream of becoming.

This is not what I expected. I thought that my garden was for bell peppers, basil, and tomatoes—payback for my efforts. It is not. In the silence of a sunny afternoon, I contemplate my impending surgery. How can I feel that yoga is worth it? How can I have faith that life awaits me within the silence of my paralysis? The answer is simple: *Because of the life in the dirt.*

After all this, it may seem that I am confident heading into surgery and in the path that waits ahead. But that is not the whole story. Simultaneously, I am past tired. My inward sense of dying, of drifting within the silence, has not disappeared. In fact, it has just barely begun to seek a healthier expression through yoga. I still long to lie down and sleep, to no longer resist the graying sensation of flying apart, of hovering above that Foster frame. The work of reentering my body seems an impossible task. In truth, I enter this surgery not entirely clear if I want to live or die.

⌐

I awake from the surgery to a voice saying, "There he goes again!" A flurry of movement envelops me. I start to realize that I am in a struggle. "Matt, can you hear me, stay with us." It is the alarmed voice of my anesthesiologist. I am in recovery and having a terrible time coming out of this lifeless sleep. My blood pressure is all over the map. Slowly, I make it back into that room, back into that body, back to a life that I am rechoosing. By the time I talk to the surgeon, I am in the clear.

His first words are, "You sure didn't behave very well." The look on his face is tired and concerned. "Honestly, I'm not sure what happened. You bled like a sieve. Have you been taking a lot of aspirin?"

"No, not anything like that." I am being told about events to which I feel absolutely no connection. I feel only a dark, grizzled humor about having returned.

"We had to give you a couple units of blood. You left quite a mess on the floor." He is shaking his head, trying to lighten the mood. "And your blood pressure, what was that about?" He slowly rubs his eyes. "There were times when it dropped off the table. I tell you, you didn't behave well at all."

"What can I say?" I smirk. I am trying to follow his lead.

"Just remind me not to operate on you next time. It's too much work." He turns and quickly heads to his next surgery. The extended length of our encounter has put him behind schedule.

I am in the hospital, but what am I healing? Is it my back or is it my past? Whatever it is, I am on fire. What should be only a three- or four-day stay turns into seven. I cannot sleep. Time won't let me; ghosts won't let me; past trauma won't let me. Each time I drift off toward sleep, there is fury. Startled, twitching, jumping, screaming—not mind, but body. I can't see it coming. Blindsided, hammered, bouncing, thudding, breaking. Then I wake to quiet, to stillness, only for it to repeat when I doze again. I am exhausted, but it won't let me sleep; whatever has me in its clutches won't let me sleep. I am overwhelmed.

I am besieged by a past that I can no longer see. I try drugs. All these years later, they now give a patient control of the IV morphine drip. I press a button and bingo. I am trying to eliminate the transition into sleep; my aim is to move straight into passed out. It doesn't work; nothing works. Something deep within me has uncorked. I am coming apart. That thirteen-year-old boy is calling me back. I am being pulled into what I left behind.

Over time, it dawns on me—I am having flashbacks. Almost all of my physical trauma has occurred between the states of wakefulness and sleep. I was dozing in the car when we slid down that embankment. I was in a coma during those first few gruesome days. I was on Valium when the screws went into my head, when they broke my wrist, and on and on. So often my trauma had come when my guard was down, when I was trusting the world, when I was taking a nap. Whether it is being in the hospital again or having my spine manipulated, my body is making me relive my past. It is gaining voice because I am finally strong enough to let it. My body has been terrified, and I am grief-stricken that it has suffered silently for so long. I can't stop crying.

This goes on for nearly three days. Barfing body memories is what I am doing. It feels completely out of my control. But the memories are helping me regain a semblance of continuity. For example, I have mentioned before that I have no memory of the day of the accident. That's not exactly true. I have no mental memory. But I am learning that my body has retained the memory; it has been holding pieces of my history until I was ready.

The experience of a body memory is hard to describe. I now know the feeling in my body when our car shot hard left as our tires hit dry pavement. I can feel the car tumble from left front corner to end over end. More than anything, I can feel the terror of traumatic time, the pause, the hanging, just before impact. (This feeling is still triggered when I am landing in an airplane and the brakes engage.) I now know that the blow to my upper thorax came from the right side at a downward angle, sweeping through my torso, from right-side ribs to left hip. I also know—from the "inside"—my shallowness of breath, my struggle for air, and my drift into shock at the accident scene. Still, twenty-five years later, if my spine moves too much or too quickly during yoga, I go into a mild version of past shock. My spine is still letting go of the echoes of trauma.

These memories are not visual. They are not thoughts. They are experienced, something like the inward feeling of falling in a dream, only to wake up just before rolling off the bed. They are pauses of fright and held in the silence before breath. They are my body bearing witness to what my mind could not.

As I lie in that hospital bed, I am temporarily living in more than one dimension of time. I did not expect this level of healing. I thought that losing the metal in my back would be enough, that this would neatly end a twelve-year chapter of disintegration. Healing, however, is not instantaneous. It is earned. There is no way to step around my body's past experience. I am terrified. My body has much to say, and it needs acknowledgment. More important, I need to feel grateful.

As I wake up to the horror of traumatically induced body memories, I am forced to feel death—not the end of my life, but the death of my life as a walking person. I absorbed death as I watched that young boy having screws twisted into his skull. The silence within which I found refuge was a level of dying.

In principle, my experience is not that uncommon, only more extreme. We all experience different levels of dying throughout our lives—the process of living guarantees it. As each day passes, especially in our later years, we become increasingly aware of our own mortality. If we can see death as more than black and white, as more than on and off, there are many versions of realized death short of physically dying. The death of a loved one sets so much in motion: grief, a sense of loss, tears, anger, a transcendent sense of love, an appreciation of the present moment, a desire to die, and on and on.

Then there are also the quiet deaths. How about the day you realized that you weren't going to be an astronaut or the queen of Sheba? Feel the silent distance between yourself and how you felt as a child, between yourself and those feelings of wonder and splendor and trust. Feel your mature fondness for who you once were, and your current need to protect innocence wherever you might find it. The silence that surrounds the loss of innocence is a most serious death, and yet it is necessary for the onset of maturity.

What about the day we began working not for ourselves, but rather with the hope that our kids might have a better life? Or the day we realized that, on the whole, adult life is deeply repetitive? As our lives roll into the ordinary, when our ideals sputter and dissipate, as we wash the dishes after yet another meal, we are integrating death, a little part of us is dying so that another part can live.

What happened to me was simply more dramatic. I absorbed an unusual dose of death at an age when I still had much living to do. Then I made it worse by working to overcome my paralyzed body. I used my will to step over it, to step over a perceived death of two-thirds of my body. My actions unknowingly injured me. Now, I can't stop crying because in this hospital I am experiencing the convulsing body of a suffering child, but I am doing so as an adult.

I am like a person choking on a piece of food—the slow motion feeling as the morsel lodges in the windpipe, the startled pause when breathing is no longer possible, the convulsive coughing that frees the blockage, and finally the watering of eyes as the peril is realized in retrospect. I have been living within that pause, a clenched stillness that grips the silence of death. The body memories are the convulsive coughs—desperate attempts to start living again. And finally the tears, the letting of water that expresses the pain of my denial.

During the previous twelve years, I have borrowed against my body. I have unwittingly relied upon the resounding beauty of its discipline against death. When I "left" my body during my traumatic experiences, it was my body that kept tracking toward living. It was my body that kept moving blood both to and from my heart. Often, as we age and can no longer do what we once could, we say that our bodies are failing us. That is misguided. In fact, our bodies continue to carry out the processes of life with unwavering devotion. They will always move toward living for as long as they possibly can. My body did not ask for the rupture that it experienced, but it somehow survived it.

I am still returning to my body and will do so for the rest of my life. I will leave this hospital with the crushing realization of my body's commitment to my living. I did not mean to take it for granted.

14

Maha Mudra

When I return home from the hospital, everything seems the same—my blue velvet chair, the sounds of my fridge, the creaking of my wood floors. Everything except for the feeling that I have recently chatted with aliens. That's how my body memories strike me. How could my body have memories? Bodies don't have memories, minds do. Not only did I believe this growing up, but my philosophical studies reinforced it. Now, in the span of a few days in the hospital, my sense of who I am, where I begin, and where I end once again has broken wide open. My body interacts with the world and records it regardless of whether my mind is having any experience.

This seems simple enough. For example, at any given time, the back of my head is visible to the world during every instant that I am awake. My body is also present in every second that I am alive, even while I am sleeping. Both of these thoughts are easy to grasp intellectually, but to feel them—that is different altogether. I felt these body memories in three dimensions. They went beyond two-dimensional mental experience and instead expressed themselves through the three-dimensional experience of my body. That my body could be a possessor of memory made me confront something that was now undeniable. My body—not just my mind—is also conscious. How does one truly open to something like this?

The act of "opening" consciousness makes us feel both uncertainty and the onrush of silence that comes with it. This is one of the reasons that becoming more aware is often painful. There are many stunning things about the Grand Canyon. One of them is the eerie silence that accompanies its vast expanse. It is both awesome and unsettling—one knows not to stand too close to the edge. The feeling of openness and a confrontation with silence are deeply related.

Opening to the fact that my body was conscious caused me intense grief. I took advantage of my thirteen-year-old body so many years ago. It was subjected to profound violence and I abandoned it in the process. Did I really need to? Was it really my only option? The existence of these body memories made me confront the silence and uncertainty of recognizing my own mistakes.

I went into surgery believing that the rods impeded my path to yoga. I came out the other side into a much bigger world, to a much bigger me. I felt like a cat who has been inside all winter and is abruptly tossed outside when the weather thaws—hunched to the ground and deeply suspicious of the immensity of open space. I had to accept on yet another level that I was profoundly injured. Worse yet, I had to admit that I was partly the cause. I needed a healing story, a way to stay grounded in this very painful and uncertain place.

I came across a Zen parable:

> A monk sits cross-legged in the middle of the road, meditating on existence. A powerful insight consumes him: He and the Universe are One. He intuits further that the Universe, being One, would never harm itself. And as long as he stays connected, he too will never come to harm. During this timeless thought, he feels the ground shaking. He looks up and sees an elephant walking down the very road on which he sits. He smiles inwardly and continues to meditate. As the animal draws closer, he opens his eyes again. A man is standing on the back of the elephant, waving his arms and yelling, "Get out of the road! Get out of the road!" Completely confident in his realization, he returns to his meditation. The elephant squashes him. As he lies there hemorrhaging to death, he calls out, "How did this happen? I don't understand." His Zen master comes out of the ditch, walks over to him, and says, "Didn't you hear It tell you to get out of the road?"

I was about to commit to the study of yoga and do so with a paralyzed body. The truth that my body possessed memory, that it was also conscious, was as undeniable as the man yelling from the back of the elephant. But I had no idea what this meant for my practice of yoga. How do you interact with a body that you cannot feel directly but is conscious nonetheless?

This story of the monk's mistake was reassuring to me. I did not need to know anything in advance. I just needed to stay open to my experience, to what was obvious. My yoga practice would talk to me like the man on the back of the elephant. I just needed to listen and not prejudge what I was being told.

This story also made me feel less alone. The Universe would talk to me when and if it was needed. My task was simple: I only had to listen. If I did, the Universe's guidance would be obvious, not hidden. I would feel connected, not disconnected. The phrase "back of the elephant" became my reminder to listen to the experience of my life and not deny it.

My lifelong commitment to yoga, my practical journey through mind-body integration, begins slowly after surgery. Not only am I sore, but this is also new territory for both Jo and me. During our first meeting postsurgery, I am still unable to do any poses. I just need to tell her about the tunnel I have been in—the hospital, the body memories, the grief. This intimacy is a testament to the strength of our relationship. Although there is already a deep connection between us, we do not know each other that well.

We are on the dojo floor—two willing students have helped me down—and Jo is sitting directly in front of me, spine erect, with the soles of her feet pressing against each other. The pose is called *baddha konasana,* and she sits in it almost the entire time we visit. Teaching without teaching.

She listens to my story, says little, and absorbs much. She intuitively knows that I have much to let go of. She knows firsthand the way memory can uncoil from a body. As I tell her about my time in the hospital, I expect the vacant eyes of polite disbelief. But instead, she nods, looks down, and whispers, "I know." Jo and I have met each other at the perfect time. My need is obvious. But Jo, too, is in transition. She is in the very early stages of starting what will become the San Diego Yoga Studio. She is ready to strike out on her own and is gaining confidence. She is also ready to take her fourteen years of yogic experience and consciously combine it with her uncanny ability to empathize with and project into another person's body. In order to teach me, she will have to intuitively connect with what it's like to be paralyzed. She will have to imagine how yoga might manifest through such a body. Luckily for me, Jo has this rare ability in spades.

So begins one of the relationships in my life of which I am most proud. There was no model for us to follow, no example from which to learn. Jo teaches Iyengar yoga, a highly refined system developed by yoga master Sri B.K.S. Iyengar. After meeting me the first time, Jo had called two senior teachers in the Iyengar method for advice. Their recommendations of one or two seated poses and some shoulder and arm stretches were of little help. She had already exhausted their ideas in our first session. She was left to her own devices, to her own creativity, to an uncommon openness that would guide our work together. She didn't have to be the expert. She knew Iyengar yoga—that was clear. I was her student—that was also clear. But we explored the possibilities of yoga and paralysis together. She made me a partner in a great experiment—the mark of a fabulous teacher.

Jo had the patience and the foresight not to force the Iyengar system of yoga onto my body. For instance, she did not worry that I could not do standing poses—the poses that are considered to be the building blocks of the entire system. Instead, Jo had faith in the system's underlying principles. Iyengar yoga distinguishes itself from other styles of hatha yoga by its heightened emphasis on alignment and precision. I believe the reason for this is profound. When anatomical structures—bones, muscles, ligaments, tendons, skin, and so on—are brought into greater alignment, the mind connects with the body more fluidly and with less effort.

This phenomenon is easily experienced. Sit in a chair, slump your shoulders, and let your neck and head jut forward away from the torso. We all know this position—we call it bad posture. Now, sit up straight, lift the chest, broaden across the collarbones, and extend out through the top of the head. Notice how presence activates in the inner thighs and down through the feet, especially through the heels. The mind moves without intent, without volition. As the chest lifts and the spine extends, the mind follows the more efficient distribution of gravity and naturally increases its presence in the lower extremities. Iyengar yoga, by emphasizing alignment and precision, maximizes this effortless form of mind-body integration. It is the beginning of realizing an energetic connection between mind and body.

Of course, this realization did not come to me all at once. I had been practicing consistently for about six months. Each morning I would get up, drink some water, and then sit in my blue velvet chair. I would take a few minutes to feel my whole body, to activate a sense of presence through my base by focusing on the weight distribution between my sits bones and imagining a connection between my chest, my tailbone, and my feet.

My actual practice was limited to four poses. I would get down on my blue exercise mats and do each pose three times. *Dandasana:* legs straight in front, palms pressed into the floor beside the hips, lift the chest. *Upavista konasana* ("wide legs"): legs as far apart as possible, hands grab the legs just below the knees, lift the chest. *Baddha konasana:* soles of the feet pressing evenly into each other, interlock the fingers, grab underneath the feet, hold them firmly, lift the chest, and stretch the torso up. *Siddhasana:* one leg bent at the knee, with the foot pressing against the opposite thigh; the other leg bent at the knee and the foot set upon the ankle of the first foot; join the thumbs and forefingers and rest the back of each hand upon each knee, palms facing upward. With such a limited repertoire of poses, I was forced to learn from the subtle differences between them. I was made to look more deeply into what could easily have become ordinary.

Just doing four poses was exciting enough. My body, paralyzed though it was, was taking the shapes of real, bona fide yoga poses. I would sit on the floor, use my arms to move my legs, bring the soles of my feet together, grab underneath them, and lift my chest. The outward result was pleasing. If a snapshot of my version of

baddha konasana were held up next to a snapshot of another beginning student's pose, they would have looked roughly the same. I
could do it.

For many students, this is as far as they delve into the heart
of yoga. They practice the poses in a strictly physical manner.
They access only the pose's outline, using their bodies to fulfill
the intended shape. For them, yoga is similar to gymnastics or
acrobatics—that is, an expression of their outer body.

In my practice, I encountered the same limitation within my
paralyzed body. When I did a pose, I would typically feel the
muscles in my upper body straining and working. But my lower
body remained essentially quiet. What cues I experienced came
from my physical position, for example, from the shift in balance
between having my legs straight and having them bent. In short,
my perception traveled primarily from outside to in.

The feeling is similar to looking at your image in a full-length
mirror. You can become so fixated on this outer image that you
briefly lose connection to the "inside" of the figure in front of
you. Perhaps you go to straighten the knee in the picture and are
surprised when you realize that it is your knee that is straighten-
ing. Now imagine living with access only to the image in the
mirror, that is, without the feeling of having your knee straighten.
In some ways, that is what it is like to be paralyzed. Moreover,
that was how I felt when I did a yoga pose—my lower body was
only an image.

But then something changed. My yoga poses gained a measure of inward, three-dimensional depth and did so without flexing muscles. A sense of energy awakened not just within my

unparalyzed body, but even more profoundly through the silence of my paralyzed body.

It was a Friday evening. Jo had made the Amtrak trip from San Diego to Santa Barbara. Upon arriving, she came over to my house. We thought it wise to check in and visit before her weekend classes began. Our work together was and is predicated in large part on our personal connection, on our ability to trust, communicate, and create in tandem. We have become wonderful friends.

The night air is laden with the ocean chill of mild California winter. Night is falling but not completely present. Lamps are necessary but not nearly adequate. Instead, there is that odd, surreal feeling as yellow light struggles against the descending darkness. My house feels little and quiet, but conversation with Jo is ripe and potent. Before long, we are on the floor doing yoga. She is introducing me to some seated forward bends—*paschimottanasana, janu sirsasana,* and *maha mudra.* I am pleased. We are doing something new.

Maha mudra is a strange pose. In yogic lore, if a yogi (yoga student) practices it enough, he or she can eat anything, even something poisonous. Regardless, it has a magical feel to it. Seated on the floor, one leg is straight in front of you. The other leg is bent at the knee, with the sole of the foot pressed against the inner thigh of the opposite leg. One reaches down, hooks the big toe of the outstretched leg with the thumbs and forefingers of both hands, lowers the chin toward the chest, inhales, and tightens the abdomen, pulling it back toward the spine and up toward the diaphragm.

As I move into this pose, something clicks or snaps into place or becomes manifest. I experience a new *ding*. I suddenly feel a tangible sense of my whole body—inside and out, paralyzed and unparalyzed. I am stunned.

"Jo, this feels different, something is different. I can feel where the pose goes, the unity between the actions. I can feel it actually moving," I gasp. "The abdomen hits back and up, and the straight-leg thigh pushes into the floor . . . right?"

"Yes." She says, breaking a smile.

"Then the . . . energy"—I struggle for words—"moves out through the heel."

"Well actually, the physical action is to hit down with the thigh and stretch out through the heel," she says, her tone informative.

". . . as the spine and chest lift in opposition," I chirp in. My mind is racing. *How am I feeling this? How is this possible?* I am perplexed, but the moment is mine. My entire body is working in concert. It has been a long time—some thirteen years. My lost body and my potential body have joined in this pose. My past, my present, and my future are touching. Although I am choking with grief, I am also an excitable boy. I have worked so hard to make it back to this moment.

Jo and I do not say much. It is too big, too fresh, and not to be spoiled. Silence—the lamp's light, the darkness outside the window, our reflections in the glass, my creaking house. My world has changed its shape tonight. A new level of me is coming alive. I am overwhelmed with the feeling that my body has been waiting for me to stop neglecting it, waiting for me to quiet down and listen. My heart is breaking. I feel grateful.

This was a simple but radical breakthrough. Jo and I discovered that alignment and precision increase mind-body integration regardless of paralysis. The mind is not strictly confined to a neurophysiological connection with the body. If I listen inwardly to my whole experience (both my mind's and my body's), my mind can feel into my legs.

This is one of those truths that is easy to pass by, like the existence of dinosaurs. But in fact, it should dumbfound us—that, on some level, something as simple as the more precise distribution of gravity can transcend the limits set by a dysfunctional spinal cord. When I move from a slumped position to a more aligned one, my mind becomes more present in my thighs and feet. This happens despite my paralysis. It is simply a matter of learning to listen to a different level of presence, to realizing that the silence within my paralysis is not loss. In fact, it is both awake and alive.

To be sure, I do not experience the same thing as most people when my mind connects within my paralyzed body. For example, as my chest lifts while in a sitting position, I cannot go on to physically press down through my heels and slightly extend my toes. I do not have the luxury of confirming my presence through flexing muscles. And yet, I still experience a level of integration. I gain some form of energetic awareness—a tingling, a feeling of movement, not outward but inward, a sense of hum. It is a form of presence, and it subtly connects my mind to my body.

This level of energetic sensation is what guides my teaching of yoga all these years later. I can teach a walking person the subtleties of a standing pose, for example, because of my energetic experience. I can "feel" the pose, feel how the physical instructions are intended to amplify, guide, and direct the flow of energy. When I teach, I give instructions and then I observe not just whether the physical actions are occurring, but also whether the intended energetic release is happening through the student's mind-body relationship. If the energy of the pose is not flowing correctly, I can often adjust the student and enhance his or her experience.

That I can teach walking students reveals something miraculous about yoga and yogis of the past. These yogis made a stunning discovery about the human metaphysic. They uncovered an energetic level of our experience and combined it with disciplined physical action. They literally made it possible for "more" of each of us to manifest Here. Perhaps most important, they were able to pass this knowledge down through generations.

My ability to sense this energetic level has greatly increased with thirteen years of yoga practice. Now, for example, if I receive acupuncture, I can often sense the changes in my energetic meridians. The needles make energy connections between different parts of my body, and my mind can often track them, even amplify them. What were once labeled "phantom feelings" are somehow related to time-tested Chinese medical practices.

The energetic realization I experienced in *maha mudra* affects how Jo teaches me. Rather than worry about maximizing the number of poses I can do, she shows me the general principles within the poses, how they actually work. For example, poses are always moving in at least two directions, usually opposite ones. Jo teaches me that there is a logic to a yoga pose, a structured way that it creates itself. This is one of the gems revealed within the Iyengar method—by emphasizing alignment and precision, poses virtually write themselves.

Up until this point, Jo and I had unknowingly assumed that my paralyzed body would be capable only of the physical outline of the poses. The hope was that I would at least derive some therapeutic benefit. For example, the soles of my feet can be made to touch each other if I use my arms to make it so. This position stretches the groin and lower abdomen and thus increases blood flow to the area—a good thing. What we didn't realize was that, once my feet were in this position and if I really paid attention, I could feel that pressing my heels together changed the awareness in my lower abdomen. This created an inner sensation of my knees moving toward the floor, which, in turn, made my lower abdominal muscles feel like they were lifting. Once this connection was felt, I could feel the sense of direction within a pose. It then became something that I could work on, something I could practice.

This has a wonderful effect. It means that I can follow the energetic flow of a pose, which allows me to see and feel the corresponding physical movements. This helps me to feel the heart of yoga despite my limited access to its physical movements. I can feel a pose's inner workings, its focus. This, in turn, allows poses, or modified versions of them, to organically arise out of the body I have, not the body everyone else has. The principles of yoga, its logic, hold for my body in the same way as for anyone else's. Its outer expression just looks different. The result is that I start to realize new ways to feel my body, to gain presence, not on the outside but on the inside. I begin to feel a different kind of life.

Jo and I part on the evening of sharing my experience in *maha mudra,* knowing that much more is possible. My entire body will be able to work on both the inside and the outside of the poses. As my paralyzed body gains strength and resilience, as my confidence in it increases, my yoga will expand to limitless places—a promise that yoga extends to any of its practitioners.

On a practical level, what begins is an acceleration of my study. In addition to Jo's visits to Santa Barbara, I travel to San Diego for one long weekend a month. A four-hour drive, a stay in a cheap motel, and an intensive focus on yoga. Luckily, Jo's family accepts me into their lives—her husband, Mike, her youngest son, Mylo, even her two older kids, Michelle and Skip, who live on their own. I do everything but sleep in their house. Mike, a wonderful cook, woodworker, and yoga teacher, feeds me and keeps me light. Mylo, the little brother I never had, I tease relentlessly—a tall order for a nine-year-old to accept. As a group, we share down-time, between time, drive time, even difficult time. I am adopted as a yoga student, a friend, and an extension of the family.

Hour after hour, Jo and I sit on her living room floor and work. Our agenda is to not have an agenda. We immerse ourselves in yoga and follow whatever comes. Before long, I am trying a new pose in a new way, and with a sense of my entire body that I never believed possible. Signpost after signpost passes behind us. Our dynamic seems to defy description. We feel part of an emerging secret, something unexplainable. Energy is moving through my paralyzed body, some sort of awareness, some sort of new life. Somehow, I can guide it, intend it, become part of it. Somehow, Jo can see it in me, feel it, focus it with her instruction. She can tell when I am not working to extend through my left leg, when my mind is only making it to my knees, or when I have forgotten my feet. She confirms what I am experiencing. I am learning to listen within my paralyzed body to a level I never knew existed. Reality is actually being re-formed for my mind.

⌒

What is happening? How is it possible? In *maha mudra*, how can I feel that the thigh hits down and the lumbar spine (lower back) lifts in opposition? First of all, both of these actions occur below my purported level of sensation, that is, below T4, my nipple line. Second, my muscles do not fire—they remain flaccid. Where is the sensation coming from? The answer is that it doesn't matter—it is coming from the back of the elephant. When that thirteen-year-old boy came to believe that the sensations in his legs did not exist, he was convinced to ignore what was right in front of him—the feelings within his own body. It's as if the monk was told by his teacher that the approaching elephant was imaginary and to pay no attention to it. Luckily, inward energetic sensation is more forgiving than an elephant's foot.

The mistake rested with the doctors. They worried that I would form a belief that conflicted with their implicit view of the potential for mind-body integration, that I would use the experience of sensation in my legs to believe that I might walk again. But there are many possibilities for healing within the mind-body relationship. There is healing other than healing to walk again.

Still, I struggled to believe that I could actually feel the inner energetic sensations in *maha mudra*. When I look at my legs, when I consider what's missing—voluntary movement, muscle tone, flexion—what is it that remains? Obviously, my legs are still physically present in the same way that a table is present. But what else? I do experience this new level of sensation, but it's not like normal sensation. It is not immediately responsive; for example, when I pinch my leg, shock waves do not instantly invade my brain. The truth is that my legs are not very interested in what surrounds them, in the texture of my pants, in the softness of my socks. Instead, they present a hum, an energetic buzz. (Imagine the buzz you feel when you finally get into bed after an exhausting day.) It gets louder sometimes, tingles sometimes, even seems to change its "color" when my legs get cold. Moreover, this buzz is directly affected by the quality of my perception, by how well I listen. Meditative attention amplifies it to the point of exaggeration; an engaging social interaction pushes it into the distant background; a rock concert makes it disappear completely.

And yet, this energetic buzz persists, fluctuates, moves, and spreads. It also reflects changes in my bodily state. For example, it becomes agitated if my bladder is too full, or if my bowels need emptying. It spikes during systemic pain, like when I have a high fever. More important for my yoga, this energetic awareness responds to my mind's intent. It becomes louder when my physical body comes into greater alignment and is "darkened" in places within my body that my mind has unknowingly abandoned.

When I look at my legs, when I truly listen, I hear what exists before movement. Through paralysis, the outer layer of my legs and torso have been stripped away. What remains is what's present before I enter the world through effort and action, before I engage my will. I begin to perceive the history of my body as similar to the fate of an artichoke as we eat it. Green leaf after green leaf, thriving muscle after thriving muscle, is peeled away until nothing but the heart remains—a heart that presents itself first as silence.

I received something in exchange for absorbing so much trauma at age thirteen. I experience a more direct contact with an inner presence of consciousness—the heart of the artichoke. Although my life has taken much away, it has also revealed a powerful insight.

This healing story also helps me relate to yoga. A new beginning for anyone's study of yoga is when the poses provide glimpses into what lies beneath their physical action. Often, it takes years of practice before this happens, before the poses present themselves as movements of energy, as an unfolding of presence. The yogi begins to see poses as expressions of this energy, not creators of it. This is what helps poses become more graceful, less strenuous, more nourishing—a heightened awareness of the energetic core of physical action. Most students' path through hatha yoga, then, travels from the physical level to a more energetic level.

My path is different. My paralysis, my life as an artichoke, gives me an early glimpse into this energetic level, the way the alignment of a particular pose creates an energetic resonance and thereby forms the whole. Once I intuit this, I attempt to trace this energetic core back into the physical and outward through my paralyzed body. In other words, I do yoga backwards. This phrase—"yoga backwards"—helps me to understand my process within yoga, helps me feel like I belong.

In *maha mudra,* I begin to realize that the silence I encounter within my paralysis is the nexus within my mind-body relationship. The silence that helped me leave my body and protected me from pain in intensive care is the same silence that helps me energetically connect mind and body. The silence can both separate and integrate—a transforming realization. In my yoga practice, the practical effect is that my paralyzed body becomes one of my teachers, not something I prejudge as a hindrance. This is healing—the potential I feel in the world breaks wide open because my realization has moved inward.

15

Broken Yet Again

In yoga, there are no accidents. Injuries are
not the result of misfortune or bad luck. They almost always have
a subtle place of origin, a harmless bad habit perhaps. But as the
bad habit is repeated, it leads to still other bad habits—cracks
appearing in a foundation. The mistake may be physical; it may
be mental. It may develop quickly; it may take years. But always
an injury can be traced to a failure in one's practice. Always the
body pays for this escalating lapse of consciousness.

The energetic realization that I experienced in *maha mudra* set
much in motion. I began to experience occasional flashbacks during my yoga practice. As I did more and more poses, especially
twists and backbends, the energy trapped in my spine began to
release. As this happened, I would revisit my traumatic past and, in
particular, the accident scene. One day I might experience rushes
of body fear—clammy sweats, shortness of breath, dizziness. On
others, I might experience a full-fledged body memory—a feeling
of falling, a collision with something, a jarring twist, the smell of
grass. Although difficult in the moment, these experiences catalyzed a new sense of freedom. Finally, the trauma that had struck

through my thirteen-year-old body was coming into my field of vision. I was surrounding it. It was no longer surrounding me.

This period of time brought some amazing dreams. I met with my sister on a landing of glass stairs. It was the meeting she had promised in four years, except it had been five and a half. I guess ghosts are not good at time. She held me, and I cried and cried. I was finally coming back alive and she was leaving me. She went up the stairs, and I slid down.

I also had an encounter with my near death. While sleeping one night, I awoke to a black presence floating just above my chest. It reached into me, grabbed my spine, and began to lift me off the bed. As it released me and flew out the window, I truly awoke, paralyzed with fear but thankful for the rising sun and the sounds of birds.

Finally, I had a series of dreams in which I kept meeting a woman. I was attracted to her, but not sexually. Each time we met, she handed me a boy to hold, beginning first with a baby and then, with each successive dream, a slightly older boy. It slowly dawned on me that these boys were versions of me. She had been caring for them until I was ready. The car accident had taken my childhood and I was finally getting it back.

This series of dreams culminated in a painful realization. The "she" in my dreams was also me—the caring, more nourishing part of me that was pushed aside when I was guided to willfully overcome my disability. For me, the integration of my mind and my body has meant realizing a deeper connection with the more vulnerable, feminine aspect of my consciousness. I suspect that the same might be true for a lot of us.

But the energetic realization in *maha mudra* also began a mistake. Experiencing this new level of energetic presence was exciting, and it was easier to feel excited than to feel how I had mistreated the "she" within me. The result was that I fell back into the clutches of an old healing story. I set out to prove the realness of this energetic sensation rather than simply have it. The result was that the excitable boy in me became very willful in his yoga practice. My body paid the price.

I repeated my rehabilitation's mistake with the silence. Rather than simply feeling the silence that contains the depth of energetic perception, I treated it as an object for my will—I pushed when I needed to soften. The result was unintended violence. I know now that energetic realization both requires and creates the realization of nonviolence. Unfortunately, I had to learn this the hard way.

I know the moment that my yoga practice passed over the threshold into violence. The pose was *paschimottanasana* (full-forward bend)—sit on the mat, legs straight in front of you; press the thighs downward, extend the spine upward; inhale, and, on an exhalation, reach down, clasp the wrist of one arm with the hand of the other and pull back against the soles of the feet; finally, rest the chin on the shins, just beyond the knees. Among a host of other things, this is an incredible stretch for the hamstrings.

I started doing this pose every day for longer and longer periods of time. This is tricky because my paralyzed body gives less feedback than an ordinary one. My muscles do not scream with anguish. This makes it easier for me to unwisely push the limits of a stretch. Eventually, however, if I really overexert in a pose, my paralyzed body will give an autonomic nervous response—its own version of screaming muscles. For example, the skin on my legs might produce goose pimples, or I might feel an energetic tingling through my bladder, or my face might flush. But this level of response is subtle. With a little bit of will, these warnings can be ignored. And that was exactly what I did. I heard my body complaining but pushed on anyway. I wanted to hold the poses longer, get their benefits better . . . faster. I wanted to prove that my body was, in fact, awakening.

One day I was showing some poses to my friend Kim. She too did yoga; it was something we shared. Because I was demonstrating, I did a particularly aggressive version of *paschimottanasana,* paying absolutely no attention to my body's feedback. She giggled nervously and said, "Wow Matt, you do that pose awfully hard." I was startled for an instant, paused, but then bristled with pride. This was the moment when I crossed the boundary.

I continued doing all my poses in this fashion. Some of the outward results were remarkable. I was doing things that defied the imagination for a paralyzed body—arm balances, various ways of approaching a standing position, poses requiring very awkward leg positions, and on and on. My body was proving itself to be quite resilient.

I was beginning to feel prideful about my body, like I had something to show. I consciously felt my whole body again when I was in a room full of people. When I talked emphatically, I could communicate with everything that I was, not just as a floating head and shoulders. My social presence became more powerful. In truth, such an effect happens for any yoga student. But for me, it was like fireworks. For the first time since the accident, I felt physically vibrant.

My budding confidence, however, began to feed my ego. I wanted more poses of greater and greater difficulty. I wanted to show beyond a shadow of a doubt that something amazing was happening within me. My poses would be the physical evidence that no one could deny.

⤻

The day of violence is June 15, 1991. June is notoriously gray and foggy in Santa Barbara. On a lucky day, the sun emerges and burns its way through the pressing cloud cover. I remember the precise day because as I get into my car that morning, I place my estimated-tax form on the dashboard—June 15. My plan is to mail it after I practice yoga in a nearby aikido dojo. (Bill and Geraldine, the owners of Aikido Center of Santa Barbara, are kind enough to let me practice in their dojo twice a week.)

Somewhat to my chagrin, Geraldine insists on being present in the dojo while I practice. She and Bill have an office in the loft upstairs, and she catches up on the bookkeeping as I work. For the last six weeks or so, I have been working on *padmasana* (lotus pose). It is a seated pose in which the left foot is set on top of the right thigh near the hip, and the right foot is set on the left thigh near the hip. Although *padmasana* is a powerful meditation pose, it is also physically demanding. It requires flexible hips, ankles, and knees, none of which I have.

On top of that, I am doing an advanced variation, one that I know now to be ill-advised. I am lying on my back in *padmasana,* legs in the air, pushing them toward the floor. The room is quiet, my breath is even, my arms are straining to push my legs away from my torso. *Crack!* A sound like a breaking branch echoes through the dojo. Everything collapses inward. My lower abdomen, my torso, my cheeks, even my skin feel pulled downward through the floor. Weight rips at the backs of my eyes. I am losing consciousness. I hear my voice in the distance say, "Call an ambulance." My vision dims. I struggle to sit up. I vaguely hear Geraldine asking in her thick French-Canadian accent, "What happened?" "Call an ambulance," I gasp. We look down at my right leg. Hanging there, held together only by skin, my femur bone is broken about four inches below my hip.

There is no doubt that most people would have been screaming. But I do not experience the same outward loudness of the gross body injury. I do not have the mind-numbing distraction of crushing physical pain. For example, I do not need the morphine offered by the paramedics. Rather, within this injury, I hear the core channel breach, the chaos of radical energetic disruption—

the breaking of a major bone. My inner body is robbed of its direction—ants swarming on honey and into the darkness of the other side. Yes, it hurts.

I am loaded onto a wooden board and placed on a gurney. The paramedic holds my leg down in a normal position so straps can be fastened. The gurney starts rolling and hits a bump. The upper portion of my thigh and hip stay straight; the rest of my leg falls off and hangs unnaturally over the edge. I experience an instantaneous loss of vision, a drastic yanking of my energy core down and to the left. I hear myself screaming.

Once I arrive in the emergency room, I am made to wait a couple of hours—alone and behind curtains—while the orthopedic surgeon is summoned. My leg is now in traction. During this time, I try to catheterize myself—I have to pee so badly—but I cannot get the catheter through my urethra to my bladder. Everything is clenched, all the muscles in my abdomen have been yanked downward. I can even feel the pull in my teeth. This remains true for nearly eight hours. By the time my body allows me to pee, there is well over a quart of urine.

Dr. Gallivan draws the curtain back crisply and with authority. He looks like Clark Kent.

"Um . . . Matthew, is it? How did this happen?"

"I was doing yoga." A sudden alertness comes over his face.

"I thought yoga was relaxing," he laughs out loud. He offers his all-American-boy smile. I tell him the details—what I was doing, my medical history, a little about the strenuous nature of yoga. I even tell him how—because of yoga—I can experience sensation within my paralysis. He patiently nods and writes stuff down. He is a good listener. I like him, but he doesn't really hear.

Dr. Gallivan is different from the doctors I had when I was thirteen. Over the course of our relationship—the next eighteen months—he demonstrates a passing curiosity about yoga, about my work, about the potential of the mind-body connection. He even considers sending his young daughter to me as a student. She suffers with severe scoliosis and is facing surgery. But this is a fact about Dr. Gallivan as a person, not about how he thinks as a trained professional.

As a doctor, he differs little from the physicians I encountered fifteen years earlier, at best displaying a change in form, not substance. For example, he does not tell me what I am or am not experiencing. He is respectful and has been trained in tolerance. Moreover, he does not give me a bad metaphysical argument, as had been done previously—that the sensations in my legs are illusory because they aren't directly physical. But Dr. Gallivan does stay stridently faithful to his paradigm, to the assumptions that underlie his medical training. He listens to my reports of energetic sensation but does not consider believing them. He does not open to deal with the particular patient that is me. Instead, I am judged to be a nice guy but also a New Age yoga nut. It will cost me.

Dr. Gallivan recommends surgery for my leg. This entails removing the bone marrow from my femur and inserting a metal rod through its entire length. Two sets of interlocking screws are then put in place, one set near my hip and another just above my knee. This procedure gives my leg the best chance of healing straight. Best of all, it means that I will not need a cast.

After surgery, Dr. Gallivan is pleased. "I got the bone back together almost perfectly. I couldn't have hoped for a better result." He is obviously proud of his handiwork. "But there is a potential complication." I freeze. I hate this kind of news. "I had to use a longer metal rod than I would have liked," he continues. "This means that the rod itself comes down to a point just above the knee joint. It puts the knee at risk to another trauma, like an awkward fall." My jaw is beginning to clench. I know this story. I've absorbed it before. I am seething with angry disgust.

"You have got to be kidding," I snap.

"But given your activity level, this shouldn't be a problem," he answers quickly. "You won't be playing football anytime soon, will you?" His humor is meant to soothe. "The good news," he says, "is that I didn't need the screws by your knee. The bone felt stable enough without them." I can barely hear him.

"What about yoga, Dr. Gallivan? What about yoga?" He looks at me, squints his eyes as if playfully sizing me up.

"Well, don't be doing lotus pose or whatever it was that caused this," he jokes. My silence makes him continue. "Seriously, you're going to have to be careful."

"For how long?" I press.

"About twelve to eighteen months, depending on how fast your body solidifies calcium." My injury is now complete.

Dr. Gallivan has made a mistake, probably one he couldn't have anticipated. He chose not to insert interlocking screws just above my knee because he wanted to save my body from unnecessary metal. I am grateful for his restraint, but he was wrong. He felt confident that I wouldn't need the extra stability because I am not a walker. What he didn't factor in is how much I use my femur bones when I transfer. Each time I lift my butt from bed to chair, they are what I land on. They are my base—the equivalent of feet for someone in a wheelchair. I need those extra screws.

I get home from the hospital on a Sunday. On Tuesday, I call his office and tell him that something is wrong. I am hurting too much. He explains this away as postoperative trauma. "Matt, remember, you just broke the largest bone in your body. It's gonna hurt." He tells me that if I'm still concerned by the time of my next appointment on the following Monday, then he will x-ray it.

I am a complete wreck. It takes me a half-hour to rally the courage to transfer into my chair to get to the bathroom. The once-a-day transfer onto the toilet to empty my bowels is excruciating. I am in so much pain, but it is not exactly pain. I am not howling or screeching in agony. Instead, I feel weak and jarred and frightened. It's like I am living in a tunnel, moment to moment, movement to movement. The pain is systemic, an inward collapsing, as if I am folding on the inside. There are times when I actually grow faint as I try to sit up. Sometimes when I move, I hear a popping sound in my leg; other times, a grinding noise. I keep telling myself, *He said it was gonna hurt,* as my vision continues to dim.

By Thursday morning, I am overwhelmed. I call his office again. This time he is impatient with me. "But what about the popping noises?" I ask. He tells me that this is probably the ligaments readjusting their position against the bone of my leg. They get quite stretched during surgery and need to reset. He tells me not to worry. "But Dr. Gallivan, this is too much pain. Something is wrong," I plead. "Matt, this isn't yoga," he retorts. "Just wait 'til Monday." He places me on the fringe. I turn back to my life and suck it up.

Come Monday, it takes everything I have to get in the car. As Dr. Gallivan puts my x-ray up against the light, the color drains from his face. He is a good man, a compassionate man. He is even a good doctor, a fine example of his medical training. He didn't believe my reports of excessive pain because he didn't believe that I could feel such things. He turns to me and says, "I am so sorry. Your bone now shows a butterfly fracture. It has been rebreaking this whole time." I inwardly hear the sounds my leg has made over this past week. I feel like vomiting.

He shows me the x-ray. The term *butterfly* describes the pattern in which my bone has splintered. "Matt, this newly developed fracture will heal just the same, just not as fast. But I have to operate again . . . go back in there and insert the extra screws by your knee." He turns back to the x-ray, stares at it, his index finger to his lips. He is running through his mental checklist, replaying his medical decisions. "Matt, if I had to do it again, knowing the information I knew when I knew it, I would have done the same thing." Incredibly, he is thinking of himself.

"You could have fucking listened to me," I blurt. I have surgery the next morning. It is outpatient surgery and I am done by midafternoon. On the drive home, I notice that the sun is shining. I can feel its warmth against my arm. Two little screws and the pain has become manageable. The relief is like landing in bed.

⌇

It is easy to point a finger at Dr. Gallivan. He could have listened better. He could have believed my reports of excessive pain and seen me sooner. With any unparalyzed patient, he would have. But the issue runs much deeper. Not enough doctors and not enough patients have turned their attention to exploring the mind-body relationship. There have not been enough patients who sense pain energetically but not quite physically—I presented a relatively new phenomenon. We don't know how a potentially deepened relationship between mind and body should affect how we administer medical treatment. Legally, I do not think Dr. Gallivan was negligent. He was following his training to the best of his ability. The problem was that the medical model itself has not transformed yet. This will take time and a lot more patients like me.

Dr. Gallivan was not the only one who failed to believe. I was the one who didn't trust energetic sensation. I was the one who was afraid to open fully to what I was experiencing. In order for energetic sensation to become real and vibrant for me, I had to let go of an old healing story. I had to stop trying to overcome the silence within my consciousness, the silence now tangibly embodied within my paralysis. This meant I had to sit still long enough to feel the silence, to accept how vulnerable it made me feel, how broken. I was not ready to feel this and instead returned to willfully proving my experience, rather than having it.

Breaking my leg was the harshest lesson that I have ever experienced in yoga. For me, nonviolence is no longer an intellectual platitude within my practice. It is an energetic fact.

16

Falling Gracefully

After the second leg surgery, it took twelve weeks for my leg to lay down enough calcium to fill in the break. It was another eight weeks before I could even consider doing yoga, and it would be a year until I could have the metal rod and screws removed. When all was said and done, it took nearly two years before I could do yoga again without exercising special caution.

During those first twelve weeks of bed rest—I could only get up to use the bathroom and get food—I had ample time to think about the direction of my life. If there was ever a time to quit yoga, this was it. I had just broken the biggest bone in my body. What other proof did I need that yoga and paraplegia didn't mix? Except that I knew better. The problem didn't lie with yoga or with my paralysis. It rested with me. I had once again misused the silence between my mind and my body. I had allowed my need to prove myself, my need to overcome my paralyzed body, to rear its head once again. The result was violence.

Rather than shy away from yoga, however, I stepped toward it. The lesson I learned about the importance of nonviolence only deepened my faith in what I was doing. Here I was, a paralyzed guy studying yoga, and the "back of the elephant" delivered a resounding message, one that was only incrementally less severe than getting smushed under an elephant's foot. The integration of mind and body requires a realization of nonviolence. Breaking my leg taught me something in the same way that my body memories opened my conception of consciousness to include my body. The lesson was not something I could deny. It was a fact of my experience.

I believe that the process of integrating mind and body teaches a person on many levels. The motivation that led me into philosophy at age twenty—the vague feeling that I somehow carried a secret about living and dying—was finally coming to fruition. When those screws were twisted into my thirteen-year-old head, my existence was spread so thin that a sinewy silence was revealed, a silence that coexisted with my living, a silence that made me stronger. It was my death.

I started to see my struggle with the silence, and my need to integrate my mind and my body, in everything around me. I began to feel it in people, in their eyes, their bodies, their struggle with purpose, and their desire to make a difference. I also began to feel it in such things as a developing environmental awareness. The environmental movement, however misconstrued, is an attempt to integrate mind and body, to balance our wealth generation and consumption habits with the body that is Earth. As I waited patiently for the return of my yoga practice, I formed the belief that mind-body integration is not just a personal health strategy, it is a potentially evolutionary movement of consciousness.

With these thoughts, the purpose of my life takes its form. I am not sure how something like this happens. For me, it is not a willful commitment. I simply wake up each morning knowing how my energy will be spent, knowing that I will explore the silence between mind and body and its connection to living. I do not have to choose it. It is what I am.

I also know to trust time. Strangely, this is something I learned while hovering over that Foster frame. Time keeps moving. It may move slowly, it may be without contour or flare, but it keeps moving, *plink, plink, plink,* as my saliva hits the metal mouth commode below. In those horrifically endless moments in intensive care, I learned how to stay faithful to living, to trust that the passage of time brings results—one way or another. My commitment to mind-body integration is timeless in the same way. If I stay faithful and keep my head down, if I work with integrity, the Universe will take what it needs. The number of years I spend doesn't matter because my faithful consistency causes time to lose its edges. This is how our kids seem to grow up in a blink of an eye.

While lying in my bed after leg surgery, I started to make plans. I imagined creating an institute of consciousness that would make the abstract nature of mind-body integration ordinary and useful. That way people would have an incentive to merge mind and body. This, in turn, would have the effect of grounding their silence more directly into their living.

I decided to move home to Minnesota. It was time for me to return. I came to California, to graduate school, looking for something, for a form of expression. I found what I needed— yoga, healing, and a sense of purpose. My work was ready to focus not just on myself but on helping others. I wanted to complete the circle and begin my work where it had all started.

Upon returning, I found that waving my hands and talking passionately about an institute of consciousness was not a very good door opener. My family and friends were happy for my return but didn't quite know what to make of my plans. They nodded blankly at my monologues and received me with open arms.

I also believed that there was a business application in what I was doing. I began to imagine a program that would help employees connect more deeply with their bodies. Not only would this program help people revitalize their sense of well-being in the workplace, it would save money for employers by curbing both rising health-care costs and workers' compensation claims. Unfortunately, what seemed to me a no-brainer for businesses wasn't quite that simple. For the time being, I had to put my imagination on hold and fondly put the institute of consciousness on a thirty-year plan.

My plans have indeed taken their time in developing. Eight years later, in 2001, I founded Mind Body Solutions, a nonprofit 501(c)(3) charitable organization dedicated to the simple notion that minds and bodies work better together. As I write this in 2005, I do a wide array of public speaking engagements, and we do have a program that goes into the workplace, called "Bringing

Your Body to Work." Mind Body Solutions also operates a yoga studio and offers workshops in the health-care field. It may not be an institute, but there are still almost twenty years left in my timeless thirty-year plan.

When I first returned to Minnesota, the grandiose scale of my ideas took a hit. The business application stalled. I did, however, join a small, fledgling sustainable investment group. The Investor's Circle is a national organization that tries to simultaneously invest in sustainable, Earth-friendly, socially responsible start-up companies while also pioneering a sustainable investment model. I continue to work with the Investor's Circle because I believe that the sustainable investment movement is itself a movement of mind-body integration. It attempts to make the generation of money more Earth-friendly, increasingly humane, more connected to body, and thus more sustainable over time.

Besides my involvement with the Investor's Circle, I temporarily put aside my plan for an institute and returned to the basics— an almost exclusive focus on my yoga practice. After a couple of years, I decided that it was time to share my experience with yoga and paralysis. If nothing else, I could help others who lived with disability. I started teaching an adapted yoga class at the Courage Center, a leading rehabilitation facility in a suburb of Minneapolis.

My idea was that by teaching this class, I could give something back—an obvious means to make my experience useful. What I found was much more. I thought I was teaching these students, when, in fact, they were teaching me. Neurological deficit is a frontier of mind-body integration. Working with these students has taught me that the principles of yoga are nondiscriminating— they can travel through any body. It has also made me honor and appreciate even more profoundly the innovations of Sri B.K.S. Iyengar. His increased focus on alignment and precision in individual poses and his use of props has made yoga accessible to anybody, regardless of their level of ability.

In this adapted class, I also get to witness the amazing ingenuity of mind-body integration. What these students are capable of, the relief that comes across their faces when they connect in new ways through such difficult bodies, makes everything else I do worthwhile. Moreover, the progress they enjoy from our working together affirms what I have learned. I teach them the subtleties of sensing energetic sensation, about moving inward and connecting through their bodies on a level that includes the silence, and it works! They experience gains in strength, balance, and flexibility. They too gain a measure of calm and a feeling of wholeness. The practical benefits of energetic realization are not just flukes of my particular experience. They apply to a wide range of abilities and disabilities.

Finally, teaching these students has shown me the different forms that healing can take. I have a student named Chris. He is now in his mid-twenties and lives with cerebral palsy. He gets around in an electric wheelchair but can stand on his feet briefly, with help. His fingers do not follow his instructions very well; his hands cannot bring food to his mouth. His tongue and speech are slowed by his condition, but not the glint in his eyes and never his laughter.

He has come to my class nearly every week for eight years, and it is for faces like his that I wonder about our limited conception of healing. It is obvious that yoga and a deepened mind-body relationship will never reverse his condition. He will always live with cerebral palsy. But can he still actively heal, not just psychologically or spiritually, but in practical ways that include his mind and body? Of course he can.

Not surprisingly, Chris needs help getting into the shower. It is a difficult transfer into a small space. Falling is not unheard of and always quite painful. When Chris starts to fall, he startles. When he startles, his body spasms, adding awkwardness to the velocity of his descent. One such fall resulted in a broken tooth.

During a class, Chris told me about a fall in the shower he experienced earlier in the week. Apparently this time, as he lost his balance and began his descent, he did not startle. He did not break into spasm but instead dropped ever so gracefully to the floor. He told me that it was because of yoga that he did not startle, that he was able to reach the ground softly for the first time in his life. Chris's eyes caught mine, and we shared a realization of freedom—the freedom to fall gracefully.

Healing can travel in so many directions, and Chris's story is not just about Chris. Barring some sort of miracle, I am never going to walk again. More to the point, my body has sustained a lot of damage, and it is never going to be easy to live in. Especially as I age, I grow more aware of my aches and pains, more aware that I have traveled through a shredder of sorts. Yoga definitely helps. It makes me feel better not just physically, not just mentally, but it helps me feel the core of my existence. Is yoga going to make all of my hardship go away? Of course not—my life is going to be hard. But without these difficulties, I would not be who I am.

If nothing else, my life has taught me one thing: The mind and body that I have are the only mind and body that I have. They deserve my attention. And when I give it, I receive so much more in return. Learning to fall gracefully through one's mind-body relationship is not a submission. One learns to fall gracefully in order to roll.

There is still so much to realize. My experience tells me that the silence within us can be experienced energetically as a nourishing sap. When this happens, consciousness changes shape. For example, I have never seen anyone truly become more aware of his or her body without also becoming more compassionate. A mental state like tolerance can deepen into a three-dimensional state of true patience. Nonviolence can become more than a moral principle, it can become an integrated state of consciousness that includes the body. And, of course, for good or for bad, the silence within us also contains the opportunity for choice.

Since my original accident, I have felt like a little boy, out of breath, trying to tell his family that something wonderful is awake in the back-hall closet. The silence we carry is not loss. It is the presence of death as it travels within us. The energies of life and death—of movement and silence—integrate within our existence to form consciousness. It requires both a mind and a body. One to open; one to stay present.

Take a moment, soften your jaw and the inside of your mouth. Close your eyes and let them sink down under your cheekbones. Let the silence spill forward and add dimension to your presence, both inward and outward. Take a gentle breath. Let it fill you up.

I have but one story remaining. It is the story that set me to writing this book. It is a story of life and death traveling side by side.

17

The Births of William and Paul

A dream healed my heart to Jennifer's possibility. It was as much a feeling as a dream—a flash of a woman walking away from me. She had long, curly brown hair and a spunky step. I was flooded with a wave of companionship, of a presence that made me playful and at ease. I startled with the thought *I can be with her.* As she walked away, I realized that I knew who she was but could not place her. I woke up frantically searching my memory but came up empty.

I re-met Jennifer at our ten-year high school reunion six months before I moved back to Minnesota. I almost didn't make it to the reunion. Two months before, I had the metal removed from my leg. If I wanted to do certain yoga poses without fear of injuring my knee, the metal had to go. I just barely recovered enough to make the trip.

I chose to be awake during this last leg surgery and have a spinal block. I wanted to confront the corrective violence directly rather than deal with its unconscious imprint within my yoga practice. I came away knowing that there is some violence for which it is better to be asleep. Orthopedic surgery is brutal. I barely was well enough to travel home and find my life partner.

Jennifer has mouthwatering eyes like chocolate-brown Tootsie Pops, is five feet tall, and has a small, angel-shaped birthmark on her left calf. She is excited by life, by plants and flowers, by photograph albums and friendship. She is constantly in touch with people and throws a great party. Jennifer reminds me of living.

I have known her since we were fourteen. I kissed her once in tenth grade, then again as a freshman in college (although she still denies the latter encounter). I would have never admitted to having a crush on her, nor she on me, but we kept coming back for more. Never quite satisfied, always sticking teasingly in each other's memory, Jennifer and I lost touch for nearly a decade.

During our first date after the reunion, she gave me a strange compliment. Jennifer was raised by a single mother. In her mind, the need for having a man around to ensure family happiness was marginal at best. She also knew that she wanted to have a child before reaching thirty—with or without a husband. A couple of years prior to our meeting again, Jennifer had lightheartedly perused her memory for men from her past who might make acceptable donors of genetic material. She cross-referenced looks, brains, and kindness. The result of this imagined search: I was her best option. Sure, I was a little banged up, but that was acquired and didn't affect the quality of my genes. As far as she knew, my family history was generally healthy.

Jennifer told me this offhandedly within the stream of our conversation. To this day, she maintains that she meant nothing by it. She only wanted to pay me a teasing but heartfelt compliment. Easy to say now. In the moment, I was a little stunned. This was not something I heard every day. I was flattered, but the timing also struck a deeper chord.

I had just had a checkup with my urologist. Since I am at risk for bladder and kidney ailments, I have one every year to get a jump on emerging problems. Unknown to me at the time, my urologist, Dr. Pryor, is a leading researcher in male fertility, particularly in the potential fertility of men living with spinal cord injuries. Three days before my first date with Jennifer, he informed me that he had pioneered new techniques in the collection of viable sperm. While I was capable of sexual intercourse and even of ejaculation on rare occasions, the quality of my sperm was unknown, and coordinating an ejaculation with a woman's ovulation possessed odds just slightly better than winning the lottery. But with his new collection technique, Dr. Pryor thought I could biologically father a child. The consultation ended with the offhand comment, "If you ever find someone you want to make a baby with, come see me."

I had gotten used to the idea of not fathering children as a defining parameter of my life. I had accepted it as part of my injury. To receive this unsolicited information caught me completely off guard. When Jennifer jokingly told me I had won her imagined sweepstakes, and I told her of my appointment three days earlier, we stared at each other and felt our lives merging.

Two years later, we were married. Our ceremony was held October 26, 1996, in the unfinished house we were building. This was the house I had been waiting for, the one I could build because of the lawsuit. It has big open spaces, vaulted ceilings, wood floors, low kitchen counters, no upper cupboards, an accessible sink and stovetop, a front-loading washer and dryer, a wheel-in shower, and an attached garage. It has an upstairs, a lift to traverse the change in elevation, a room dedicated to yoga, and best of all, it is on a lot full of beautiful, old maple trees. Building a life of love and laughter with Jennifer has landed me fully into my life. Eventually, we will even make babies.

William Matthew and Paul Loren were conceived through in vitro fertilization. Jennifer and I did not have an easy time of it. We had six inseminations. That meant six surgeries under a fast-acting general anesthesia for me. Three of those times, Jennifer was given hormones to increase the odds, and six times, even with optimal placement of my sperm near her eggs, we were disappointed.

Finally, the doctors suggested in vitro fertilization. For reasons unknown, her eggs and my sperm were having trouble getting the job done. In vitro fertilization gave us a friendly boost. The process was far from easy, however, especially for Jennifer: lots of hormones, an egg harvest, a petri dish conception, and an implantation. The first time failed.

After our second attempt, Jennifer was sure it hadn't worked. She was having what she thought were menstrual cramps, and we were having a garage sale. When the dreaded call came, she was sitting behind a card table, counting odd change. Her eyes popped wide open in disbelief. She was pregnant. For three years, fertility issues had been looming over us, a period long enough to take on a life of its own. Suddenly, the process was over and another had begun. Our surprise was genuine.

⤳

During our first ultrasound, the doctor calmly said, "How many kids did you say you wanted?" Jennifer was pregnant with fraternal twins—two separate embryos. There we were, a girl five feet tall and a boy in a wheelchair, and we were having two babies. Jennifer turned to me and said in a voice that mixed fear with joy, "Why can't we do anything normal?" We left the ultrasound and went out to an unplanned lunch. There was silence and laughter and hand-wringing and long exhales. We kept telling each other a healing story: "Well, it may be more work up front, but we can be done having kids now." Two children were as many as we wanted. "Look at it this way—we are getting two for the price of one." In vitro fertilization is not cheap.

By definition, having multiple babies involves higher risk. We were sent to a specialist in high-risk pregnancies, but he did not expect any problems. His plan was simply to monitor the pregnancy more closely than usual. We experienced quite a few ultrasounds.

We gave our children their names early on. William Matthew,

the baby usually in the lower left section of Jennifer's belly, presented his gender early—at about fourteen weeks. Suddenly, there
he was, all boy and facing outward. A few weeks later, Paul Loren
followed suit, as Jennifer watched the ultrasound screen in disbelief. As an only child raised by a single mother, she had always
imagined having a girl—she knew nothing else. On top of that,
we had recently gotten two boy kittens from the same litter. By
Jennifer's count, that made five boys and one girl in the household
of her future. Her initial dismay turned to laughter and then to
love as her life kept changing before her eyes.

Although Jennifer's presence makes her seem tall for her size,
twins in her stomach were quite a stretch—literally. Each night, I
would rub vitamin E ointment into the skin of her exploding
belly. This was my time to give, both to her and to my two sons.
I would tell William and Paul stories about their mother, about
our life together, about the life we would all share. There are
many reasons why a pregnancy lasts nine months. One is so there
is ample time for a family to dream of their life together. This was
one of our strong suits.

In retrospect, Jennifer and I can now recognize the first signs
of trouble. At night as I rubbed her belly, Jennifer would give me
a report on our sons' activities: "William had hiccups again
today," or "Paul was awfully rowdy this morning." Over time,
however, she noticed a difference between the two. William's
personality felt softer, quieter. This mirrored my experience when
I put my hands on him. One day, as Jennifer was giving her
nightly report, she referred to William as her sweet child, and
Sweet William became his name. We imagined how this early

difference between William and Paul might manifest in their personalities. Each night, as Jennifer and I listened to William's emerging silence, it innocently lit our imaginations.

Our routine ultrasounds had become greatly anticipated—another opportunity to see the boys. That all changed when, out of nowhere, fluid appeared on William's brain, a condition called hydrocephalus. This development was surprising because we were already thirty-two weeks into the pregnancy. Problems of this kind typically appear much earlier. The doctor assured us that the condition is not usually fatal. There are four ventricles in the developing human brain. They are a reservoir system for the flow of spinal fluid. If there is a slight variance between input and output, the fluid accumulates. The brain's tissue, then, becomes oversaturated, causing damage. The severity depends upon the amount of fluid that accumulates, which in turn depends upon the discrepancy between input and output.

The causes of hydrocephalus are many. Any kind of blockage could be the culprit, ranging from a microscopic defect to a clot to countless others. The doctor's strategy was to let the pregnancy move forward unchanged—the safest place for William and Paul remained in their mother's womb. After the birth, William would probably undergo a procedure to insert a shunt. Basically, a drainage tube would be surgically inserted into the problem ventricle. The long-term prognosis was impossible to know—being dependent on far too many variables. The only things we were consistently told were that William would most likely live, that there was no obvious risk to Paul because they were fraternal twins, and that William would probably have some disabilities—both mental and physical—the extent of which was unknown. Jennifer and I watched as another possible life passed us by. It was the week after Christmas, and we had to make plans, not just for a new year but a new life.

Upended is how we felt. But we were parents, expecting new life into our midst. Jennifer was planning and grieving and protecting all at once. Her Sweet William was going to have surgery on the second day of his life. How was she going to breastfeed him? Where was she going to stay? Where would Paul be? Never underestimate the pragmatic strength of a mother protecting her children. This was one of the first of many examples that I would witness.

My work was on a different level of our future life—the integration of a "special" child into our stream. While Jennifer was preparing to land our boys into the world, I was whispering to William. I was telling him that he could not have landed in a better place, that I too lived with a disability, that I had spent years realizing a different path, a more integrated one. I told him that I was a yoga teacher and he was my best student, that our work—if he desired—could traverse a lifetime. I would help him live vibrantly through whatever mind-body relationship he was dealt. I told him that he had given my life new purpose—I would now work primarily with kids. Finally, I whispered that I was proud to be his father.

William's presence in my life felt like the back of the elephant. I had been wondering how to bring meaning to my path, how I could give back. Suddenly, my work at the Courage Center took on new significance. My experience with people living with all sorts of disabilities, including a couple of teenagers with hydro-cephalus, now felt like preparation. It felt like the Universe was deepening my commitment to helping people with disabilities—rather than being part of what I do, it was to be the main focus. I was surprised by this, but also relieved. My path was clear. There was no way I wasn't going to help my son live as gracefully and magically as possible. Best to make the rest of my work congruent with that commitment.

On a personal level, William's looming disability also injured my heart. One of my jokes to Jennifer during the course of her pregnancy was, "Do you think my sons will come out in little wheelchairs?" So wonderful was the feeling that the struggle in my life would not be passed on. Most likely, my sons would walk through their entire lives, stand while peeing through their entire lives, have spines that would remain unbroken through their entire lives. So freeing was the thought that the car accident would finally end—at least physically—with the advent of my next generation. To have a son who would share my struggles was crushing. It felt like a continuation of my life's rupture. It did, however, focus my purpose.

Each night during the two weeks after the diagnosis, I would rub Jennifer's growing belly and talk to my whole family. My life had taught me that there is a wealth of strength within us; there is nothing we cannot handle. Life presents its purpose and beauty in all sorts of ways. The trick is to stay open to one's strength, to not deny or strive to prove it, but rather to simply have it. I told my family that we would be fine and our lives together would be an adventure. But to William, especially to William, I silently whispered that I was ready, that he should come, that everything would be okay.

When William died in utero at thirty-four weeks, our lives were upended again. The planning, the purpose, the research, the healing was suddenly for naught. Jennifer and I were awash in silence, in grief, in a spin of painful emotion. We looked at each other, moved closer, and did what we always had—made the best of what's around.

The path ahead was completely unknown. Jennifer was carrying our dead son inside her body. Next to him was a vibrant, kicking, playful little scrum who was living, eating, and resting his head next to his dead brother.

William's death did not change the medical strategy. The best place for Paul's continued development was still in his mother's womb. Because William's slowly disintegrating body posed little threat to his brother's well-being, the doctor's plan was to monitor Paul closely and head off any potential problems. The pregnancy went forward on a natural course. William would deliver first because he was positioned lower than his brother. His birth would be like any other, except his body would manifest the completion of death. Paul would follow, and we would finally meet our two sons—one living and one dead.

This scenario was impossible to enter in advance. Despite the horror and the imagined revulsion of greeting death through the birth of a son, it was impossible not to be excited. Jennifer and I were having our babies, and its promise carried us forward.

We spent the three and a half weeks between William's death and the birth of our sons trying to prepare for what was unimaginable. Each night, I still rubbed her belly—which was now becoming lopsided as William's body was leaving us—and talked to my family. I told Paul that I admired his spunk, his hiccups, his occasionally kicking feet, his general charm. I kept whispering to William, wondering if this was his choice, wondering if he had been afraid, and praying that he was finally at peace. My hands were not afraid to feel his dwindling body. I longed for it, for any contact with my departing son.

Most of all, I watched a mother carrying her babies. I experienced the pauses she encountered as she told her story to people around her, the hushed tones: "You mean you're going to carry 'it' to full term?" or "You mean there's nothing they can do?" I watched as William's name disappeared from our social dialogue, as people didn't intend to be injurious but were, nonetheless. I watched a mother whose driving instinct was to follow Paul, but whose aching heart reached back to honor William. I watched her healing story emerge, a commitment. If at all possible, William was to receive a vaginal birth, an introduction into the world like any other child, an affirmation of his presence in our life. Jennifer's motherhood would include him in every sense in the extraordinary event of birthing.

Jennifer has strength that even her closest people often fail to see. It is a silent depth that gets overshadowed by her excitement about life, by her wholehearted desire to be a part of it. She carried a dead baby for nearly a month; she protected her other baby with everything she had. Most important, to this day, she loves her birth experience. Jennifer showed me in the clearest terms our human commitment to living, how a mother's drive to produce life can surround even a dead son. To this day, I remain honored to have borne witness.

Labor began at about ten in the morning. We called Paige, a sassy, redheaded Texan who was to join us on our journey. Paige is a mother of three—all birthed at home—two of whom are twins. She has a down-home woman's wisdom about her, and Jennifer wanted her wisdom in the room. I needed it, too.

She came to our house and we spent the day together. We played Yahtzee and cards and watched a movie. We timed Jennifer's contractions, Paige helped her take a bath, and I pressed my hands upon her lower back as each painful wave struck. We acted as a seamless team.

About eleven that night, Jennifer's water broke. The fluid pouring out of her body was brown. Paige and I said nothing, but panicked with the worry of meconium in the amniotic fluid. If a baby empties its bowels in its sac, it creates a toxic environment that can be life-threatening. Jennifer sensed our concern and, through the haze of her accelerating labor, told us not to worry—she somehow knew that all was fine. The brown water turned out to be from William's sac. We were encountering the first signs of his death.

Her assurances, however, did not help the nearly thirty-minute ride to the hospital. Neither did the fact that Jennifer's contractions were just over two minutes apart. As I was checking Jennifer into the birthing ward, I looked over my shoulder to an image I will never forget—Jennifer, propped up by Paige's sturdy presence, her body beginning to heave her dinner. With tears of love in my eyes, I paid homage to her fierce determination.

Things were moving fast. After Jennifer quickly got settled in a bed, I realized I had to piss like a racehorse. Thankfully, the bathroom in her room was accessible, and I started to catheterize myself. I kept going and going. When I was just about finished, the doctor came in to check on Jennifer. From the bathroom, I heard him say, "Better start pushing, William is on his way." There I was, in the bathroom with my pants down, and my son was being born. No use feeling bashful, I rushed out into a room full of people. I literally watched William's birth with my pants down. It seemed fitting somehow.

One, two, three pushes from Jennifer, and William is out. His body is small, only three pounds and two ounces. He looks so little in the doctor's hands. His eyes are closed and his arms are crossed over the front of his body. I do not see particulars. I see only my son, the one that decided not to come. Jennifer looks and smiles as her tearful eyes hand him silently over to me. Motherhood pushes her on. She has another baby to birth, and it will be a long night. William is my charge now. In some ways, I think he always was.

This is the moment I cannot anticipate. What will it feel like to touch my firstborn? William is wrapped in a blanket and handed to me. This has been such a long road I have been traveling. I am rejoining the group at yet another level—by entering an ageless club of proud fathers. Yet my passage is through death. The paradox, the struggle of my life comes fully to bear. This is the moment where the silence in me could have broken in either direction. I am vulnerable, I am lost, and I am in love, all at once. As I bring William against my breast, my life is being defined. He is warm . . . how could he be warm? How could death be so beautifully warm? I look over at his mother, lost in the work of delivering her next boy. It is she. It is her love that surrounds our child. She has been giving and protecting his life even through his death. I feel a mother's strength, but also our humanity. We are living, loving creatures, traveling through both life and death. Our drive for light permeates even the dark. In this moment, I have never been so in love with life . . . and so unafraid of dying. Life and death are not opposites. They are partners in the same belly.

In a twin birth, it is best for the second to happen quickly after the first. Apparently, as the time between births grows, so does the risk to the second child. The good news is that Paul is definitely on the move across her belly—like a fish just barely surfacing. The movement of the skin on Jennifer's stomach marks his travels. The doctor informs us that this behavior is not uncommon. Twins share cramped space. Take one out and it's a party in there. We watch Paul basking in his newfound freedom. Then the contractions hit; the walls of his palace close in around him, but he is undeterred. Paul continues his roaming.

The night wears on. Jennifer's labor stalls. Despite Paige's magic tricks and the labor-inducing drugs, the contractions never reach birthing velocity. Paul just won't present in the birth canal. He is having too much fun.

Not so his father. Despite my communion with William, my fear of death still lingers in the room. I need this other boy to live. Paige and Jennifer know everything is fine, but I need confirmation. Hour after hour passes. I move between holding William and fixating on the monitor following Paul's heartbeat. William is taken away briefly, given a bath, and returned to our room swaddled in blankets. I begin to have doubts. In the early morning, I detect a smell. I am horrified and crushed. I turn to Paige and say, "Maybe William should be taken away. I think he is beginning to smell." Paige asks the nurse to leave briefly and comes to me, crying and smiling. "Matt, that is not William you're smelling. The nurse has really bad BO." We break out laughing. Jennifer joins in, as she has been struggling with the nurse's smell all night. Lifted from my hole, I go over and pick up William and kiss his little head.

At ten the next morning, the doctor recommends a cesarean section. We are relieved. Jennifer is exhausted, and we need Paul to join his family in the outer world. Enough with clinging to your mother, I tell him.

As the father, I am present during the C-section. Jennifer is given a spinal block, so she is wide awake. A surgical screen separates her head from the rest of her body. I am positioned at the juncture so I can see the surgery and talk to Jennifer while making eye contact. At one point, I am literally watching the doctor's hands pulling out her guts when Jennifer turns to me and says, "You know, I could really go for a cheeseburger." I am now witness to the greatest moment of mind-body disconnection that I will ever experience. The only possible reply I can muster: "That's my girl."

In only a moment's time, I watch Paul being pulled from Jennifer's belly, his cry becoming audible like sound emerging from a tunnel. He is beautiful and healthy. I watch him have a brief newborn physical examination while Jennifer is sewn back together. He passes brilliantly and is taken to get cleaned up. I hear Jennifer's command, "Don't let that boy out of your sight! Bring him to me as soon as you can." As I ride up in the elevator with Paul and the nurse, I am the proud father of two.

Later, William and Paul and Jennifer and I are physically in the same room for the only hours we ever will be. I am struck by the calm, the beauty and ease with which we are a family. Paul in Jennifer's arms, William in mine, we are happy as we drift off into the silence of sleep.

Paul is almost four now, and the office in which I write this book is a studio built across our driveway. I hear the garage door open and his feet lightly hitting the pavement. It is through the silence that I feel him approach. I am both outside with him as the crispness of October touches the sweetness of his face and inside typing hopeful words into the dulling glow of my computer. As his pace quickens up the wooden ramp, I feel his presence enter my body. It is the strings of silence that connect us, like strands of stretching taffy. He is the continuation of life, and I am grateful for the opportunity of living.

The door opens. "Papa, when are you coming in?"

"In a minute," I say.

Paul walks sheepishly across the floor and stands next to the desk drawer with the Life Savers in it. As he plops a piece of candy into his mouth, his brown eyes sparkle. "It tastes good, Papa!" The silence within me smiles because I know that he is right.

Afterword

I

Life and death traveling as partners in the same belly—an experience that we have shared through the story of the birth of my sons. It is not just my story, however. It is an energetic truth that is occurring right now in this moment. You are living and dying simultaneously. This is the story of our aging consciousness. It is both the beginning and the end. It is a paradox of our existence and it gives me reason for hope.

Life and death, silence and action, emptiness and fullness at the same time—these are inward features of everyone's life. They are truths that do not lead to answers. Instead, they invite us to believe in and appreciate our own experience. When we do, when we carefully listen to what we experience, the next story begins, the practical one, the story of what happens *beyond waking*.

II

What moves a person to action? After the birth of William and Paul, something shifted in me. Up until that point, I had been diligently practicing yoga and teaching an adaptive yoga class at the Courage Center, but my mind-body musings had remained abstract and philosophical. This was a means of self-protection. I was willing to *tell* other people about the nature of minds and bodies, but I lacked the strength to share my personal awakening, to make my insights come alive. That changed when William's body was warm, when Paul's crying became audible, like sound emerging from a tunnel. There are moments in life when it becomes necessary to do something more, when strength is no longer the question, but only what needs to be done. I needed to let my experience be the teacher. I started to write *Waking* in the month following the birth—March, 2000.

The problem was that I didn't really know how to write, at least not something people would want to read. I was trained to write as an analytic philosopher, but knew nothing of telling a story. For the most part, analytic writing is stripped bare of beauty and description. It employs rigid language as a means to hold down abstraction. The value is placed on creating an impersonal voice that can convey a sense of objectivity. It is useful for its purpose, but does not typically lead to a page-turning story.

In those first months between March and June of 2000, I fumbled around writing what is now Chapter Two—waking up from my coma and the description of the accident scene. I also wrote a whole chapter that is now reduced to the opening sentence of Chapter One—about my nickname Jolly. These writing experiences were enough to convince me that I needed further instruction. I signed up for the first Duluth Writers' Workshop at the University of Minnesota Duluth, a nine-day course in the town of my childhood. There were three independent sections in this workshop: poetry, fiction, and memoir. Ironically, I signed up for the fiction section. My reasoning was that I needed to learn how to tell a story. Apparently, I still hadn't grasped that I needed to tell *my* story and not someone else's.

As luck would have it, the fiction section was cancelled. The workshop organizer convinced me that, given my submitted sample of writing, I would be better off in the memoir section. This is how I met Patricia Francisco, my writing teacher, first editor, and now close friend. Patricia is the person who showed me how to fall in love with writing. I particularly remember two conversations early in our relationship. In one of them, Patricia told me that I was "a ripe piece of fruit and my story was long overdue." With these simple phrases, she let me know that I was ready, and that I had a story worth telling. She also gave me a gentle sense of urgency—my story should ripen no more.

In another conversation, Patricia began what would become a mantra both from her and to me: "Matt, you need to step forward into the pages. You owe it to the reader." With this line in my head, I could sense when I was protecting myself, when I was trying not to feel. I am a private person and *Waking* is a very intimate book. While writing, I kept pushing myself to stand in front of my words and not behind them. To whatever extent *Waking* is effective, it is because of a hard-earned willingness to share: share not what I wanted my story to be, not what I thought it should be, but what my story *was*. I needed to share it without judgment, without protection, and without sentimentality. I needed to trust and believe in my experience.

This advice is not just for the writing process. Stepping into the pages of your life, finding the stories that propel you forward is an essential step beyond waking.

III

How does one transform the experience of loss? One of the steps is to recognize it as a mind-body sensation, not simply as an end. Try the following:

> Take in a breath, hold it, keep holding it, hold it a little past what is comfortable. Feel the silence. Notice the shrinking feeling you have on the inside, the silent but acute end of your inhalation, the abruptness, the trapped feeling like there is no place to go, the beginning of anxiety, of desperation.

This is what it is like to wake up to paralysis. This is the abruptness of loss experienced like the wall at the end of your inhalation. Remember that time when your arm fell asleep so badly that you could neither move it nor feel it? The startling silence in that unresponsive limb rendered you powerless. But now try something different:

> Sit up straight and tall. Feel your sits bones on the chair seat, feel your feet resting on the floor. Feel the back side of your body, the ribs behind your heart, feel your

feet again, this time a little toward the heels. Soften the skin on your face, your jaw, your temples, and especially the inside of your mouth. Take a couple of gentle breaths.

I imagine that this felt nourishing, like a reprieve. As in the first example, this too is the silence. It is feeling that underpins the experience of loss. But in this second case, it has become a mind-body sensation, a living sensation. It has been subtly integrated with the alignment of your body and the added dimension of your breath. The silence now feels like a part of you and not just a brick wall.

This is the story I told in *Waking*, the story of walking from a well-lit room into a dark one. Instead of holding my breath and pushing my way forward, I paused, stayed patient, allowed for stillness, and waited for my eyes to adjust. I kept breathing, and started to work with the darkness (silence) rather than against it.

When I did, when I listened to the silence of my paralysis and allowed it to become a mind-body sensation in its own right, a different world appeared, one with greater depth and potential. My experience of loss became not an end but an energetic truth, an aspect of my mind-body relationship rather than a breathless limit. This transformation deepened my sense of presence and connected me back to the world. It made me feel lighter, especially in my spine. My movements became more graceful, more effortless. My balance increased, my ability to listen and share with others increased. My world shifted from inside to outside.

IV

I carry an insight that transforms the experience of living with a disability. It is simple; so ordinary that it is easily passed over: The experience of presence within the body is a precious gift— a secret to living well. I know this because I lost it through trauma, at least I lost the main vehicle for experiencing it—a fully functional central nervous system. What I now know is that presence within the body can and should be approached from many directions. This is crucial for everyone, but particularly someone living with a disability. When one explores alternative methods of gaining presence, a lightness appears, especially throughout the spine, bones, and joints. This lightness is not accessible through strictly physical action—it takes something more. It also has practical, everyday benefits—improved mobility, quality of breathing, motor planning, ability to manage stress. Perhaps even more important, this lighter feeling of presence brings a new sense of freedom and hope, a new feeling of potential.

Presence, however, is a loaded word, a hard notion to grasp but something pretty straightforward. Try the following:

> Slouch in your chair, lean back, and let your knees splay out. Notice what you feel in your legs, the feeling in your feet, the dullness running through your midsection. Notice this as the feeling we often associate with relaxation.
>
> Now try moving from this position to sitting upright. Put your feet squarely on the floor and directly below

your knees. Feel your sits bones on your chair seat, broaden across your collarbones, and balance your head over your neck. Notice that as you moved forward into an upright position, you began to feel your legs more, even your inner thighs as your feet connected more consciously with the floor. Take a breath and notice how much more you feel within your body.

Simply put, this change in the quality of your inward sensation is what I mean by presence. When mind and body intersect, the result is the *sensation* of presence. Refining and expanding this level of sensation in every way possible is essential for someone living with a disability. Gravity already feels extra-heavy for us. A feeling of lightness within the mind-body relationship is more than a convenience. It is a form of healing.

I believe honing this level of sensation transcends the experience of living with an obvious disability. It holds promise for all of us. After reading *Waking*, I hope this becomes clear.

V

Visions grow from the center outward, not in a straight line. Only recently did I fully realize that the center of my work began in 1997 when I started teaching the adaptive yoga class at the Courage Center. Something wonderful was happening in that quiet, unassuming, yet spectacular Monday night class. Good, caring people—both students and assistants alike—gathered week after week and pioneered new territory. We opened the transforming experience of yoga for a population that all too often gets left behind. Moreover, we developed the mind-body insight that promises to transform how our health care approaches rehabilitation.

I also received something for which I am deeply grateful. I have seen firsthand that our groundbreaking work did not require a flash of genius. It required only trusting time, ordinary week-after-week time. That thirteen-year-old boy who hovered over the Foster frame in intensive care learned something that this forty-two-year-old writer still works to appreciate: Time brings the result—all that is needed is an intuitive sense of direction and a sense of purpose. These, of course, come from recognizing the patterns and stories of one's life, like a river gaining current. Fortunately, it doesn't take genius. It only requires paying attention.

Teaching this adaptive class has also made me practice sharing both my own loss and feeling loss in others. It prepared me to write *Waking* and showed me how to traverse a path of helping: I am no longer afraid of my own suffering, of my own grief. I know that it will come, that it will pass like a cough, that it will return, and that it will pass again. I realize that this will happen for the rest of my life.

The adaptive class has made me hopeful about the transformative potential of connecting mind and body. Mind-body integration heals on many levels at once—mental, physical, spiritual, psychological, and emotional. Perhaps most important, it also reveals the subtlety and practicality of energetic truth.

I founded the nonprofit organization Mind Body Solutions in

2002 as an extension of what I was exploring at the Courage Center. I had the notion that I wanted to work not just with disabled people, but also with the "abled." We opened a yoga studio to help people experience the benefits of connecting mind and body. I created a workplace program called *Bringing Your Body to Work*. This, too, came right out of the adaptive class. I realized that the issues facing people who sit at a desk all day aren't that different from someone who sits in a wheelchair.

Now, in 2008, the new mission of Mind Body Solutions is to transform trauma and loss into hope and potential by awakening the connection between mind and body. This mission feels like coming home—both a relief and a little scary. A relief because all the threads are finally coming together into a coherent knot. Scary because it is an ambitious vision.

First, we plan to develop curriculum and training so that an adaptive yoga class can become standard at rehabilitation facilities across the country. We are also beginning a two-part documentary film project. In the first month of 2008, we began work on a ten-to-twelve minute short film. This is intended for patients and their families who are living through trauma and loss. We want them to know that a mind-body approach will positively impact long-term outcomes. This shorter film is the first step in making an hour-long documentary.

In the second month of 2008, in partnership with the Courage Center, we began a pilot program to infuse a mind-body approach into all their rehabilitation processes. This is also a research project to collect the outcomes that will help other institutions believe in, and eventually implement, such an approach. Imagine a health-care system where it does not take twelve years to begin to reconnect mind and body.

All of this is preparation. In 2009, we aim to create a mind-body program for returning veterans. The trauma and loss of these men and women must be met head-on. I know we can help. I also believe that the necessary support will come to us when we are ready. I trust time and have faith in the goodness of people. Finally, I also know that each day I am one day closer to creating an institute of consciousness. Perhaps we will call it *Waking*, perhaps not. What I do know is the general direction in which I am heading. These are my steps *beyond waking*.

VI

Since *Waking* was published, I often find myself in rooms with readers, adding my body, my greenish-blue eyes and speckling grey beard to the story under discussion. In many of these rooms, I encounter a similar question, "How do you keep smiling? . . . How, when so many others do not?"

This question always gives me pause. I want to give a clear, resounding answer because the questioner is looking for a secret and I so want to give it. But I am unable because I do not know. I usually respond with what I already offered in this book: "I was born with a smile on my face." Of course, this leaves an unsatis-fied taste in both of our mouths. It leads to an obvious retort: "What if someone isn't so lucky? What then?"

Today, as I am writing, it is a sunny, blue-skied winter day and I am willing to try a different answer, a different healing story. My answer today is, "Blame it on the sun." Or how about "Blame it on my sons." . . . for they amount to the same thing. Earlier in this book, I wrote that, "I am both heartbroken and desperately in love." I was mistaken. I have never been heartbroken. It is not possible. What I thought was broken was actually my heart revealing its depth. It has affinity not just with having and holding but also with silence and loss. It has affinity not just with living but also with dying. Hearts are transcendent. They do not break, minds do.

We are living and dying simultaneously . . . and we are given time to realize the lightness that accompanies this truth. It is the beginning of the journey. It is the end. If I still need a reason for smiling, then blame it on the sun.

Paul is almost eight-years-old now. He has a mop of thick, brownish-blonde hair. His eyes are brown—not quite as scrumptious as his mother's, but deeper, darker, and with a sparkle that moves the earth under my feet. Paul wonders about his brother, more this year than in years past. Sometimes, right before bed, I hear him ask Jennifer about William. As our collective heart aches, I hear Jennifer pause briefly in the darkness of his bedroom, and then kiss him lightly on the cheek. In this moment, we all step more deeply into our lives.